PRAISE FOR JUST BREATHE OUT

"The BreatheOutDynamic system goes way beyond oxygenating red blood cells."

Radu Kramer, MD
Integrative Nephrologist
Bergen County, New Jersey

"Betsy Thomason demonstrates the importance of the strength of the outbreath in maximizing performance, and leaves no one out, in terms of addressing this concept. You will also learn to use rhythmic breathing to monitor effort—a key ingredient to self-awareness. This book will prove extremely useful for the layperson, professional, and college student alike. I highly recommend the techniques outlined in her book for anyone who exercises."

Susan M. Tendy, EdD
Retired Physical Education Professor
United States Military Academy
West Point, New York

"The BreatheOutDynamic system is worthwhile because it is perfect technique."

Lee Coleman, MA
Professor Emeritus, Physical Education
Whitman College
Walla Walla, Washington

"Reading *Just Breathe Out* and practicing BODs has been incredibly transformative for me personally and professionally. A vast number of my patients have disordered breathing and sympathetic nervous system dominance — causes of a vast array of health complaints that are epidemic in our society. BODs is cutting-edge therapy that treats the root cause of these medical issues. The longer I practice medicine, the more I realize that health is dependent on proper breathing."

Steve Henke, MD
Board-Certified Holistic Family Physician
Fort Collins, Colorado

"Breathing out thoughtfully, as represented in *Just Breathe Out*, is the concept that links BODs to yoga, west to east, new with ancient. As a pathologist, I can tell you that the balance of oxygen and carbon dioxide in human tissue affects every chemical reaction in the body, which in turn affects all mental and physical abilities. Betsy Thomason's sincere efforts focusing on the outbreath will help all people, but especially those with respiratory illness."

Madhulika, MD, DCP
Consultant Pathologist, Yoga Practitioner
Hi Tech Pathology Lab
Roorkee, India

"Breathing regulates our body's internal autoregulatory system—the autonomic nervous system—that maintains homeostasis and cellular function. This whole system is of paramount importance for healthy living. *Just Breathe Out*, a comprehensive review of optimal breathing techniques for health, demonstrates the involvement and power of breathing in this autoregulatory system. I commend Betsy Thomason for her valiant effort in completing this book."

Ramesh Adiraju, MD, FAAC
Founder and President
RENU-CA Autonomic and Endovascular Research Institute
Bristol, Pennsylvania

"Ms. Betsy Thomason, thank you for teaching me how to breathe."

Salihou Djabi (1945–2015)
Imam, Community Activist, Prison Chaplain
Brooklyn, New York

"In *Just Breathe Out*, Betsy Thomason has compiled a collection of careful observations and inspiring stories demonstrating how the age-old practice of coordinating breathing with activity can open up new worlds of understanding, performance, and pain management."

Josiah Child, MD, FAAEM
Chairman, Emergency Medicine
Los Alamos Medical Center
Los Alamos, New Mexico

"*Just Breathe Out* is a clear, concise guide to breathing and living better. The BreatheOutDynamic system has enriched my life, both physically and spiritually, in countless ways. As a coach and priest, I recommend you read *Just Breathe Out* and incorporate BODs into your daily routine."

Ed Hasse, MDiv
Priest, St. Paul's Episcopal Church
Physical Education Teacher, Fieldstone Middle School
Montvale, New Jersey

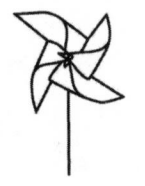

JUST BREATHE OUT

JUST
BREATHE

Using Your Breath
to Create a New,
Healthier You
OUT

BETSY THOMASON, BA, RRT

Foreword by Mike Ramsay, MD
Chairman, Department of Anesthesiology
and Pain Management
Baylor University Medical Center

North Loop Books

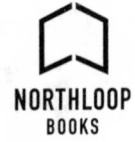

NORTHLOOP
BOOKS

North Loop Books
322 First Avenue N, 5th floor
Minneapolis, MN 55401
612.455.2294
www.northloopbooks.com

ISBN-13: 978-1-63505-334-0
LCCN: 2016910785

Distributed by Itasca Books

Cover Design by Mary Ross
Typeset by Anna Kiryanova
Illustrations by Alice Goldsmith
Editing by Ruth Thomasian

Author's website: www.justbreatheout.com

Printed in the United States of America

DISCLAIMER

Just Breathe Out: Using Your Breath to Create a New, Healthier You is a health care book based on ancient wisdom of the outbreath. It is designed as an adjunct to your health maintenance routine, not as a replacement for medical care.

Remember, some breathing problems are more related to the heart than to the lungs. Consult your medical professional to identify the cause of a problem so that you can take appropriate action.

DEDICATION

Ann Lane Mavromatis (1933–1986)

Occupational Therapist and Extraordinary Human Being

I thank you for helping me through a blocked intersection of my life. When your life was waning, you breathed life into mine. You introduced me to BreathPlay, as it was known then, which helped me through the rough spots in life and kept me focused on what was important—becoming a respiratory therapist. Ann, you gave me my life's work. And I'm still climbing mountains.

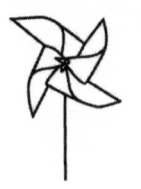

DEDICATION

Ian Jackson (1943–2011)

Womb, Heart, and Mastermind of BreathPlay/the
BreatheOutDynamic system; author, *The BreathPlay
Approach to Whole Life Fitness*, Garden City, New York:
Doubleday, 1986

Ian, I thank you for trusting my interpretation of
your work and considering me a partner in the expansion
of your mission. You granted me your blessing to use
your breathing approach in my life's work and to use my
own ingenuity when teaching it. Your spirit continues to
inspire my endeavors.

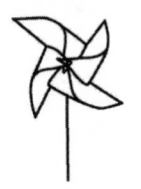

ACKNOWLEDGMENTS

I have so many people to thank—family, friends, medical and education professionals, patients, and even strangers in need of new approaches to well-being. I really understood the importance of writing *Just Breathe Out* when a third grader who had just made a pinwheel told me that BODs would help him "manage stress."

I am indebted to Sabrina Prewitt, widow of the late Ian Jackson, for recognizing *Just Breathe Out* as an authentic interpretation of Ian's work.

Alice Goldsmith, artist/illustrator, translated my words into line drawings that bring BODs to life. My twin sister Ruth Thomasian guided our editing partnership for five years. Ruth's mentor, editor Polly Hovsepian, offered her expertise with early drafts of the manuscript. Julia Muino; Richard Losh, RRT, JD; and Wylie Hembree, MD, edited *Just Breathe Out* from a medical perspective. My teenage grandsons, Jesse and Daniel Harris, read an early version of *Just Breathe Out* and even found some goofs. Many of the folks who requested the prepublication *Just Breathe Out* pdf, including Anne Hurwitt, Dave Livingston, Brian McRae, Susan Slewa, Jean Fox Czaposs, Penny Peed, Dano Carbone, RRT, and Victor Wrobleski, offered their thoughts as well. Thanks to all for sharing time and talents.

I credit the title *Just Breathe Out* to good vibrations with my neighbor and graphic designer Patty Catanzaro, also a wordsmith. We were walking and talking, and she was pushing me to get to the essence of my passion for teaching breathing. "Well, it's so basic," I said. "All you really have to do is . . . just breathe out."

In 1989, the Newark, NJ, Fire Department — Chief Lowell Jones and Deputy Chief Alfred Frieda — welcomed me to train members of the hazardous materials crew, to study the effects of efficient breathing on their use of self-contained breathing apparatus. I am so appreciative of the chiefs' interest in exploring an innovative approach to the well-being of their firefighters. In 2011, at the invitation of the American College of Chest Physicians, I presented this research at CHEST, the college's annual conference. I am ever grateful for the college's recognition of the importance of this research.

When I was a breathing trainer without RRT after my name, the late Allan M. Levy, MD, one of the original sports medicine docs and team doc for many New York professional teams, asked me to coach a professional basketball player as well as a West Point plebe, both of whom had anxiety issues related to their physical abilities. Dr. Levy's confidence in my ability to help people over hurdles affirmed the importance of the BreatheOutDynamic system. Thanks, Doc.

In the mid-1990s, when I was in charge of the pulmonary rehabilitation program at St. Barnabas Medical Center in Livingston, New Jersey, my eighty-year-old patient, the late Herbert Silberner, MD, told me that despite his pulmonary fibrosis (stiff lungs), BODs was the reason he was able to continue playing tennis. His enthusiasm helped move me forward at a time when I needed a medical doctor to confirm that I was on the right track.

While at the 2007 birthday party of my home care patient, Lucy Koch, I met her husband's daughter, Debbie Koch. During our brief conversation, Debbie asked me, "When are you going to write the book?" I started that night. I was a stranger to Debbie. She felt the importance of BODs just from our conversation.

My outdoor activities, which combined work and play thirty years ago, led me to BODs, impacting my ability to really enjoy vigorous activity, even to this day. To my hiking and cross-country ski buddies and to members of both Adventures for Women and Ski for Light, thanks for connecting the importance of effective breathing with having fun outdoors.

BODs is now a large part of my work life. During my twenty-plus years as a respiratory therapist, so many people have encouraged me. I thank Mary Ellen Downey, CRT, and Donald Downey, owners of Millennium Respiratory Services, Whippany, NJ, my employer from

2000 to 2016. I'm grateful to Steve Scelsa, MD, director, and Daniel MacGowan, MD, codirector, of the Mount Sinai Beth Israel Amyotrophic Lateral Sclerosis Clinic, where I participated on the ALS Team for thirteen years and shared my innovative respiratory therapy.

At the 2014 annual Congress of the American Association for Respiratory Care, I introduced myself to keynote speaker Mike Ramsay, MD. His address was titled, "First Do No Harm—Patient Safety & the Role of the Respiratory Therapist." He discussed prevention of preventable deaths caused by mismanagement of pain medication and the role of the respiratory therapist to prevent errors. True to the title of his keynote address, he listened to my brief BODs pain remedy and instantly said, "Yes," when I asked him to write the foreword for *Just Breathe Out.* Thank you, Dr. Mike Ramsay, for putting your body and mind into your foreword.

I give thanks to the following doctors for expanding my knowledge base, substantiating the validity of BODs, and hanging in with me for the long haul: Josiah Child, MD, pediatrician and emergency room doc; Selma Calmes, MD, retired anesthesiologist; the late Forrest Bird, PhD, ScD, MD, mechanical ventilation pioneer; Ramesh Adiraju, MD, cardiologist and autonomic nervous system specialist; Gerald W. Deas, MD, MPH, MA, preventive medicine and community health expert; Lisa Zacher, MD, pulmonologist and occupational health doc; Radu

Kramer, integrative nephrologist; and Gordon Larson, MD, retired ophthalmologist.

To all the people who have attended my breathing workshops over the years or experienced my spur-of-the-moment training, thanks for being open to the revolutionary, life-changing idea called BODs. I'm grateful to the people who have shared their BODs experiences, both anonymously and bylined in *Just Breathe Out*. Your stories enrich us all.

The publishing community at North Loop Books mirrored my passion for *Just Breathe Out* from their perspective as editors and human beings. I'm appreciative of their patience and guidance during the publishing process. I am so proud of our work together producing *Just Breathe Out*.

CONTENTS

FOREWORD

We breathe all the time, from birth to death, when asleep or awake; yet in normal circumstances we are rarely conscious of our breath. The automatic rhythm of breathing arises in the respiratory center in the brain stem at the base of the skull. The nervous system carefully regulates breathing to maintain optimal oxygen, carbon dioxide, and pH levels. Our very existence depends upon breathing. It is a key component of sound production—speaking and whistling are only possible by controlling expired air flow.

In general, we consider inspiration the active component, and expiration the passive component of breathing. We are all familiar with the command, "Take a deep breath." It may be used as a stress control method or a mood changer when emotions are getting out of control. It is a conscious, slow inhalation.

Just Breathe Out promotes the exact opposite— focused exhalation. Perhaps the only outbreath most of us ever do is after a stressful moment when we breathe out with a "phew" and think, "That was a close call."

Author Betsy Thomason helps us rethink how we breathe—from the usual focus on breathing in to how to focus on breathing *out*. It's called the BreatheOutDynamic system, or BODs, for short. Thomason uses her clinical skills and knowledge as a respiratory therapist and her understanding of anatomy and physiology, plus her own insights into mind and body interplay, to further develop the BreatheOutDynamic system, which was initiated by Olympic cycling coach Ian Jackson in the early 1970s. BODs challenges our whole concept of breathing and how we do it. *Just Breathe Out* seeks to improve our understanding of the dynamics of breathing and its importance for our overall well-being.

I have been an anesthesiologist for forty years and have controlled the breathing of thousands of patients undergoing major surgeries, such as liver, heart, and lung transplantations. The breathing focus in the operating room (OR) has always been on inspiration created by a mechanical ventilator to ensure that both lungs are inflated properly during surgery. In my OR experience, there is really very little thought about expiration, unless there is wheezing or air trapping. During lung transplantation, it is always such a thrill to see the surgical clamps come off the new, donated lungs as I slowly and gently reinflate the organ that had spent the previous four hours in an ice chest. The lungs come to life, expanding to fill the open human chest—a wondrous sight. The ventilator is switched on and connected to the patient's airway. The new organ expands and relaxes like the wings of a manta ray. In the OR, our focus is on gentle inflation and observing the lungs rise up in the open chest. We would only be concerned with expiration if the lungs did not empty properly.

So the BreatheOutDynamic system—with its focus on breathing *out*—challenges my forty years of medical practice. It has made me rethink all my ideas about breathing. Adjusting to active expiration leading to passive inspiration takes time. When I started using BODs, it did not feel natural to me. I had to apply my mind to a process that up to now had been mindless. BODs takes me into a different zone and makes the clinical scientist in me start to think about the physiology of this change in focus.

I remember my early physiology training and the famous *Textbook of Medical Physiology* by Arthur C. Guyton. The author uses the term *vis-a-tergo*—a pushing, accelerating force—to describe the movement of blood to the heart from the extremities of the body, a force generated by *expiration*. Now, I use this logic to think about the movement of air in the human body. As we expire air from our lungs, a negative pressure, or suction, develops in the chest cavity, which is then used to passively draw air back in during inspiration. This force will also pull venous blood, depleted of oxygen, back into the chest. This force from behind—*vis-a-tergo*—applies, I realize, not only to blood filling the heart and then being pushed into the capillaries surrounding the lungs, but also to movement of gases in the respiratory system. This movement of air and blood makes it possible for the lungs to unload carbon dioxide and pick up vital oxygen that will keep every cell in the body energized and ready to perform its job. When I think of it this way, it all starts to make sense.

The idea of focused breathing is to put us in touch with our bodies. Thomason invites the reader to develop a user-friendly body with the BreatheOutDynamic system. When I first read these words, I didn't stop to think about them. Breathing is good, I thought. Therefore, if we can improve how we breathe, that will bring more oxygen into our cells, enhancing their function — that's good for our bodies. Is that what "user-friendly body" is conveying? No, I don't think so.

As I thought more about it and studied Thomason's writings, there seemed to be more to this concept of a user-friendly body. To study it further I entered into my own BODs program. I started by spending thirty minutes first thing in the morning working at the active process of breathing out. Now it is so alluring that I find myself sitting in lectures actively breathing out. While working through the BODs process, I started to use muscles that I have only been conscious of in the gym — my abdominal six-pack: rectus abdominis, a pair of muscles commonly called abs; external and internal obliques; and transverse abdominis. My spine awakens and gets involved. Suddenly, there is a whole symphony of activity that my body likes. But is this the user-friendly body? Maybe part of the way, but there has to be more.

Now, weeks into my BODs program, I realize that I am a little more lithesome — I can bend a little easier — and a spring has come back into my step. Is this just mental, or a real physical improvement? I think that it is both and that the user-friendly body includes mind, spirit, and activity. It's the body that will do what you ask of it, without complaint.

I love books that challenge me with new, life-changing concepts and ideas. Does the outbreath really put you in touch with your body? Is this yoga, a mental-focus exercise, or an awakening of spirituality? I suspect BODs involves all of these components and maybe more. Like you, the reader, I'm giving it a try, and becoming hooked. I find myself sitting in an airplane, immersed in the breathing-out consciousness. I am oblivious to the cramped space and the seat-back in front of me that is almost in my lap. My back has stopped complaining. My body has stopped complaining. I have found my user-friendly body.

In this book, Betsy Thomason takes us to another level of physical and mental performance that improves both physical and cognitive functions. *Just Breathe Out* makes BODs available to all who want to improve their well-being. I am sure that you will be motivated to *Just Breathe Out.*

Mike Ramsay, MD
Chairman, Department of Anesthesiology
and Pain Management
Baylor University Medical Center
President, Baylor Research Institute
Dallas, Texas
April 2015

INTRODUCTION

Just Breathe Out: Using Your Breath to Create a New, Healthier You helps you, the reader, learn an empowering breathing system that gives you the opportunity to develop a user-friendly body. We've all heard about user-friendly computers. Now you're going to learn to develop your very own user-friendly body. The BreatheOutDynamic system (BODs) is a refreshing and profound way to take charge of your health with a readily available source of information and self-motivation—your incredible body. Think of me, the author, respiratory therapist Betsy Thomason, as your guide on this journey.

BODs, the core of this book, is the revolutionary breathing method designed by Olympic cycling coach Ian Jackson. He questioned everything and welcomed challenges as a means of gaining inner peace. BODs benefits all human beings, regardless of age or physical status. It is out-of-the-box thinking at its best. It redefines breathing from sucking air in to pushing air *out*.

But you ask, "Why is it necessary to change the way I breathe? The whole world has been doing it for so long, and it seems to work."

Here's why. Breathing is actually the process of

breathing *out*, not in. The outbreath energizes and relaxes the human body. Who knew? Well, ancient yogis knew but reserved this wisdom for the military and those with money. Now this information is available to all, just for the modest price of this book.

BODs maximizes well-being because every cell in your body relies on the oxygen you breathe for its existence and intelligence, and because breathing efficiency equals effectiveness. Since most of us rely solely on our *unconscious* breathing process for oxygen nourishment and carbon dioxide elimination, we have lost touch with the benefits of effective, focused breathing. Thus, our bodies have become dumb. The diaphragm—the most important muscle of respiration—no longer knows how to work.

Optimal health requires movement. Movement of muscle and bone is part of the breathing process. Moving through our environment is supported by breathing. But body movement is undervalued in our modern culture, as reflected in our homes, schools, workplaces, and communities. We are glued to the television or cell phone 24/7; we drive our kids to and from school where gym and recess are being eliminated from the curriculum; and neighborhood children are not playing outdoors after school. At work, most of us sit in chairs all day.

As a result, most people's breathing is rapid and shallow, leaving the body pleading to take in more oxygen and get rid of more carbon dioxide. But the body's pleas are not addressed because we do not understand their meaning, and our muscles are weak. Or if we do hear the pleas—cramps, chest pressure, low energy, depression, pain—we're not sure what to do. We have come to accept dysfunction, resorting to drug use and surgery, even pleading with doctors for prescriptions for antibiotics to treat the common cold or cough.

The BreatheOutDynamic system, with its focus on the active, spine-stretching outbreath, enhances your ability to listen to your body and trust it. When BODs becomes part of your daily routine, you will feel energized and relaxed at the same time. You will start to understand your body's messages. As you learn to rely on your outbreath for strength during daily exercise, you'll be tapping a new source of inner peace. The net result is a deeper appreciation of your body, clearer thinking, and improved physical stamina. The time you spend learning BODs and moving your body is not lost or wasted; rather, time is returned to you through improved efficiency and insights all day, every day.

Life is about continual change. BODs is the tool that makes positive, healthy change possible with every breath you take. It changes the way you think about the breathing process, challenging the assumption that breathing is an *in*-out process. When using BODs, you turn the breathing process upside down, making breathing an *out*-in process.

Are you ready to rely on age-old understandings about the design of the body, gravity, and changes in air pressure? Do you desire a more comfortable and functional body? Are you willing to allocate time every day for your own health care?

If you *are* ready to orchestrate your own well-being, this book is for you. Everyone benefits from learning to breathe more effectively. BODs is a living metaphor. When you expend energy, you get it right back. When you blow air out, the same amount returns automatically. BODs is surprisingly uncomplicated and basic. It is also surprisingly complex and beautiful.

OVERVIEW OF *JUST BREATHE OUT*

SECTION 1 THE BODs BUZZ

Chapter 1 **Inspiration from the Outbreath**
      BreatheOutDynamic system *Stories*
      Find yourself in these stories, written by BODs beneficiaries, and feel their excitement.

Chapter 2 **Building the Case for the**
      BreatheOutDynamic system
      Proof Is in Your BODy
      You'll discover the results of BODs research with elite cyclists and firefighters, and learn from information gathered by observation and personal experiences.

SECTION 2 THE BODS BASICS

Chapter 3 **Learn the BreatheOutDynamic system**

The Two-Step Basics

Right off the bat, you'll feel a calm engulf your body. Then you'll be hooked. BODs will change your life and how you view the world. So be prepared.

Chapter 4 **How Your BODy Works**

Rethinking Breathing

Take a tour of your body's airway to identify structures and their functions and discover the connection between breathing and how other parts of the body work. Knowing why BODs is so effective is an important motivator.

SECTION 3 FITTING BODS INTO YOUR LIFE

Chapter 5 **The Next Step**

Using BODs with Movement

The BreatheOutDynamic system is more than just out-in breathing. Ian Jackson developed the rhythmic recipe that helps you determine how much air you need to comfortably accomplish specific tasks.

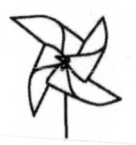

THE BODS BUZZ

CHAPTER 1

INSPIRATION FROM THE OUTBREATH

BREATHEOUTDYNAMIC SYSTEM STORIES

"Winning is the most important thing in my life, after
breathing. Breathing first, winning next."

George Steinbrenner, principal owner
of the New York Yankees

AUTHOR'S PERSONAL EXPERIENCE

*J*ust *Breathe Out* redefines breathing from a focus on
breathing in to a focus on breathing out. BODs shows
you how to honor your body and make it user-friendly.
The result is harmony between mind and body.

In this chapter you will read about real people
developing their BODs skills and how those skills
have affected their health and well-being, and added
to their coping skills. Of course, I, too, am a student of
the BreatheOutDynamic system. I use the present tense
because my learning continues every day. BODs is an
essential part of my daily exercise routine, which is

always changing depending on the season, my mood, and what adventures I'm planning. BODs not only keeps me in shape, but also rescues me from tight places.

In 2005, I was doing physical therapy to restore the use of my left shoulder, which had frozen because I had tumbled down a hill sideways while cross-country skiing. During this hour-long torture three times a week, I clung to BODs. Without the active, spine-stretching outbreath, I would not have been able to push myself to increase the repetitions of exercises. Nor would I have survived the pain of the process of "ranging" during which the physical therapist manipulated my frozen shoulder to expand its range of motion.

My self-imposed task during ranging was to stay totally focused on BODs. As long as the physical therapist was moving my arm and shoulder, I was involved with my outbreath. I was right there *in* my shoulder helping it to relax and open up. It was painful, even with BODs. The benefit of my BODs focus was increased relaxation and thus my ability to manage pain. As a result, I was able to complete the therapy; whereas, the therapist said, "Many people cry 'Uncle,' give in to the pain, and give up on therapy." BODs got me out of a tight spot, just in time for the next ski season. Today, my arms and shoulders are stronger than ever because I continue to exercise them.

AUTHOR'S PROFESSIONAL OBSERVATIONS

At work, the BreatheOutDynamic system is my magic wand. It is patient-centered therapy; that is, it empowers the patient. Using and teaching BODs, I stay focused on what's really important — self-help — not pity, lectures, or depressing test results.

A large part of my work as a respiratory therapist is helping people with breathing issues related to neuromuscular weakness, such as muscular dystrophy, polio, and amyotrophic lateral sclerosis (ALS). I help my patients adjust to ventilators that breathe for them. But no machine — even the ventilator — lives up to BODs ability to foster your development of new skills, insights, and well-being.

Here are a few of my professional observations. I've changed the names of my patients to protect their privacy.

Billy and his wife Viola, both in their seventies, came to the ALS clinic at Mount Sinai Beth Israel Medical Center in New York City for a consultation. During my 2001–2014 tenure as staff respiratory therapist at this weekly clinic, my official job was to test patients' lung function. To do this job with heart and soul, I added BODs instruction, even though I only had a moment or two for teaching. With Billy, I quickly demonstrated the BODs basics. Then I showed him how to organize his actions in three distinct movements to rise out of a chair more easily.

(See illustrations 6.6c and 6.6d.) First, he exhaled as he moved his butt to the edge of the chair and let in air. Second, he exhaled as he leaned forward with his shoulders over his knees and again let in air. Third, he exhaled as he rose to his full height, smiling with satisfaction at this renewed ability, despite his weakened legs. Knowing that caregivers also expend lots of energy, I asked Viola to use BODs to rise out of her chair. On her first try, she too expressed excitement at the ease of her efforts.

I first met eighty-year-old Armen the day he returned home from a few weeks at a rehabilitation center where he had been recuperating after being hospitalized for a week with congestive heart failure. He had experienced several heart attacks, had a pacemaker and defibrillator implanted in his chest, and was using a ton of medications. He had physical therapy at the rehab center, but said no one ever mentioned effective breathing.

When he was discharged, I was assigned to set up his home oxygen concentrator. He used supplemental oxygen via nasal cannula (an easily removable tube) twenty-four hours a day because he could not keep his blood oxygen saturation (SpO_2) above 88%. (Saturation of 97% is normal; anything above 88% is acceptable.)

Armen was not happy about being attached to oxygen around the clock. He had places to go and was still driving a car. When we went into his kitchen to sit at the table, he removed his cannula, as if to say, "I don't need this when I'm sitting." I decided to teach him the BreatheOutDynamic system immediately. When I placed a pulse oximeter on his middle finger to monitor his oxygen saturation, it registered 85%, low enough to require supplemental oxygen. As soon as he got into a BODs rhythm, his SpO_2 climbed steadily into the mid-90s. It even hit 97% briefly. During my ninety-minute visit, he continued to use BODs intermittently. While sitting focused on BODs without supplemental oxygen, his SpO_2 remained in the mid-90s, and his respiratory rate was in the normal range of 12–20 breaths per minute.

This outcome delighted Armen because now he could relax, knowing that using BODs would help him lead an active life without being constantly tethered to an oxygen tank or concentrator. He understood that he had to be committed to learning and using BODs to maintain an adequate SpO_2.

I noticed that when he walked to the bathroom, even with oxygen, his breathing rate increased to more than 30 times a minute and his shoulders started to rise toward his ears, indicating shallow, labored breathing. We discussed the importance of focusing on BODs, even when using oxygen, to reduce his work of breathing. He expressed understanding that with daily BODs practice, he could train his belly muscles to activate his strength-giving outbreath. Thus, Armen began to participate in his own health care. ❀

The summer I taught BODs at asthma camp, eight-year-old Jimmy was one of my students. He asked me if you could have asthma in your legs. I had never been asked this, nor had I ever thought of it. I was grateful for his question. It showed the depth of Jimmy's body awareness and ability to think out of the box. He understood that air does more than simply enter the lungs. Oxygen has to reach every cell in the body, and carbon dioxide must start its journey to the outside world. When Jimmy walked, his legs felt heavy and burdensome. He learned the BreatheOutDynamic system that week at camp but was reluctant to attempt a hike in the woods on the last day. After some cajoling, he gave it a try. Jimmy was able to complete the half-mile walk in the woods without heavy legs. Truly, that's expirational and inspirational.

FIRST-PERSON ACCOUNTS
WRITTEN BY REAL PEOPLE

KAREN BROWN
Retired registered nurse
and medical device rep

As a young child, I had polio, a neuromuscular disease that destroys a large part of the nervous system. The body does a miraculous thing: it tries to replace as many of the damaged cells as possible. In fact, these replacement cells actually allowed me nearly normal function for decades. Those of us who survived polio learned to conquer whatever was in our way and never show any weakness. Eventually, however, these weaker replacement cells begin to burn out. With the resulting muscle weakness, function begins to decline, pain returns, and the ability to conquer fades. This is the beginning of post-polio syndrome.

Now I am in the post-polio phase. Over the years, my breathing muscles became so weak that I had no defense against microorganisms. I am not able to fully oxygenate my blood. After a debilitating bout of pneumonia, I started to use a breathing machine during sleep.

Betsy Thomason was the respiratory therapist who set me up with a ventilator with a nasal interface (noninvasive, requiring no intubation). And she introduced me to the BreatheOutDynamic system. Since I have embraced BODs, I have been able to connect my body, mind, and spirit through this simple act of focusing on the outbreath. It's amazing that something that you must do to live—breathing—can be therapeutic! When I practice BODs, it's time for *me*, time to refocus on what is important, whether for relieving pain, controlling muscle spasms, negotiating stairs, or just putting the brakes on life. I do not know what is around the bend in my life, but with BODs in my muscles, I feel ready.

In early 2015, I experienced total skeletal muscle collapse related to dysfunction of my autonomic nervous system and was hospitalized for five days. With spasms in my chest wall muscles, I had to focus on the outbreath. This way, I wasn't fighting the spasms. The inbreath was so painful that I couldn't even tolerate my ventilator because it was pushing air in, stretching my muscles, already in spasm. I can truly say that BODs outbreath saved me. Now many months later, having recovered, I feel clarity of mind and connected to my body. And, my lungs are better than ever. 🔆

ED HASSE
Priest, physical education teacher,
long-distance runner

In the Judeo-Christian tradition, it is believed that all human beings are infused with the breath, the spirit, the life of God. "And God formed the human of dust from the soil, and God blew into its nostrils the breath of life, and the human became a living being" (Genesis 2:7).

As a priest, I have incorporated the BreatheOutDynamic system into my morning routine of prayer and meditation. Sitting quietly and concentrating on breathing out and in for five minutes enables me to find deep relaxation, rest, and openness—a sense of transcendence. Simply concentrating on actively breathing out and just letting air in, I am able to ignore outside distractions and gently brush aside interior thoughts when they bubble up, helping me to be open to the spirit of life within me. After several minutes of quietly using BODs, I find myself refreshed and renewed for another day. BODs fits perfectly together with Psalm 46, as I interpret it: Breathe out. "Know that I am God. Be still." Let air in.

As an athlete, BODs has helped me to improve my running and swimming and to push my physical limitations. I have run twenty-four marathons and many shorter races, including triathlons. Since learning BODs, I have been able to relax my body and mind, enabling me to work with less effort in times of high exertion—like my seventh New York City marathon in 1999. Ah, that Queensboro Bridge into Manhattan at mile 15! The bridge is a one-mile steep incline just past the halfway point. Everyone's energy reserves are beginning to wane, but the finish is more than ten miles away. As I approached the bridge, I refocused my BODs rhythms. Concentrating on my outbreath enabled me to power up the steep incline and maintain my personal-best pace.

During a marathon, exhaustion and pain are inevitable. It is in this state of extreme exertion and fatigue that BODs helps me most as I breathe out any cramps, pains, mental fatigue, and doubt, and let confidence enter effortlessly with the inbreath.

FRANK GLASSON
Trumpeter, cyclist, dad

After fourteen years of bike racing in the highly competitive San Diego region, I was bumping up against my performance ceiling. Not wanting to accept that, I searched for help and found Ian Jackson.

I spent some time on Jackson's website. [Editor's note: website is no longer available.] I was impressed. The BreatheOutDynamic system was definitely different from what I'd heard from conventional coaches. In a nutshell, Jackson was turning the breathing process upside down. Instead of sucking air in and letting it out, I'd be pushing air out and letting it in. I'd also be using a gearbox of rhythmic patterns to coordinate breathing and movement across the full range of work rates. Each active outbreath would tap the power of my stretching spine.

So I spent two weeks of bike riding focused on BODs. I was so pleased with the results that I decided to put BODs to the test on the 5,500-foot climb up Mount Palomar. My best time on this climb had been 1 hour and 45 minutes — Category 3. The best time for a Category 1 racer, or pro, was Chris Horner's 51 minutes and 15 seconds, to win the Tour de California in 2011. To my amazement, this time I was at the top of Mount Palomar in 1 hour and 10 minutes. This level of improvement — 35 minutes — seemed impossible after only two weeks of BODs training. A few days later, I returned to Mount Palomar to try the climb again, this time paying special attention to my watch to make sure that I had it right. To my further amazement, I was at the top in 1 hour and 5 minutes.

I called Ian Jackson to tell him my story and get his feedback. He was happy for me, but clearly not surprised. As a matter of fact, he pointed out that my BODs skills were very rudimentary, that I was only scratching the surface, and that I had much to look forward to.

And he was absolutely right. BODs continues to enhance my cycling and make me competitive. I spend less time training than the best cyclists. BODs makes my work playing the trumpet much easier and improves my stamina. What I like best about BODs is that it closely resembles the skill sets required to be a good musician: focus, confidence, and curiosity to seek more knowledge. Now I use BODs all the time, even carrying my three-and-a-half-year-old son. BODs makes life more enjoyable. 🍃

FREDDIE KELSO
Retired banker, teacher,
lover of the outdoors

It's a pitiful situation when you can't breathe. Sometimes, the only way I can breathe is to lean forward with my shoulders hunched toward my ears. I've had the symptoms of asthma since I was a kid in the 1930s.

One recent winter, I had pneumonia three times. I was homebound for a while and felt trapped. The only comfortable position was sitting, doing nothing—not my style. I'm an outdoors person.

In the 1990s, I discovered Betsy Thomason and Adventures for Women (AFW), which offers women training in outdoor skills. The BreatheOutDynamic system was part of the training. During one memorable AFW outing, I was the slowpoke, but I discovered that BODs gave me power to walk farther than I could have imagined, with less fatigue. It has given me the courage to continue my love of canoeing. A few summers ago, I enjoyed paddling on a lake in the Adirondacks. BODs was my partner with every stroke.

When I walk, I always use BODs. As it is, I can only stand up straight with great difficulty. Over the years, I have developed the bad habit of leaning forward to improve my breathing and my balance. BODs allows me to walk more effectively with less forward tilt.

Now I coordinate BODs with my daily exercises. This is key to my well-being.

JEN DIORIO
Teacher, playwright, thinker

When I attended the BreatheOutDynamic system workshop in early 2008, I was full of anxiety about work and life in general. My chest was tight, my body was even tighter, and my breathing was stifled. As the workshop unfolded, the simple words of instruction — words that asked what I knew about breathing, what I expected to get out of this breathing workshop, and what I dreamed about doing — calmed me down. Merely focusing on my breathing reduced my anxiety. What a relief, I remember thinking, I am learning something that will help me relax.

As Betsy shared the BreatheOutDynamic system, at one point drawing an analogy with a bellows, I had an epiphany. I remember being at the library, reading about how to breathe from the diaphragm, but without anyone there to show me, it was just an easily forgotten exercise. Betsy's use of simple props and her gentle requests that we get actively involved in the process made a big difference. Putting my hand on my belly, visualizing the bellows, and paying attention to the movement of my abdomen toward the back of the chair forced me to focus, slow down my body and mind, and breathe more efficiently.

Walking and using BODs was initially a challenge, but in no time I developed a rhythm, one that made me feel connected to my body and the entire breathing process, one that cleared my mind because I was no longer focusing on my worries.

By the end of the workshop, I felt like a new person. In fact, I looked like a new person also. How do I know? Well, I remember going to the restroom before the workshop and looking at myself in the mirror. I looked stressed, and my stress was in my face, which is where I carry it more than any other part of my body. After the workshop, I went back to the same mirror, and my face looked bright, happy, and relaxed. It was amazing.

Focusing on BODs lets me replicate that new-person feeling—in the morning before I get out of bed, in the car ride to and from work, and during a tough day. When I am using BODs, my entire day just goes so much better. 🎡

MICHAEL ISAACS
Psychotherapist,
wellness coach

I discovered the BreatheOutDynamic system twenty years ago when I attended Betsy Thomason's workshop in New Jersey. At that time, I was a full-time lawyer and a part-time yoga teacher. We networked and talked about our common interest in breathing for health, energy, and relaxation. At the basic BODs workshop, I learned the power of exhalation and how the active outbreath promotes an effortless inbreath. I have incorporated BODs imagery into my own teaching because it assists my own learning process.

Over the years, I transitioned from law to psychotherapy, from teaching yoga to teaching *t'ai chi chih*. Personally, I practice BODs daily. Whenever

I become aware of my muscles tightening up or my breathing being shallow, I take a brief BODs break to alter the situation and bring myself back into balance. I might be in the car at a red light, or waiting in a bank line, or at airport security, or in the waiting room of a health care provider.

One of my favorite times to practice BODs is while walking. Soon after I rise in the morning, I start my day walking either indoors or outdoors. Usually, my count is 6 steps on the exhale and 3 steps on the inhale. BODs gives me a surge of energy when I'm walking. I remember the hills of San Francisco where I used to live. BODs sure beats coffee and steroids!

When my energy is depleted, using BODs is a natural way to revitalize my system. Often, I do it lying down on my back for relaxation. In this position, BODs has helped me overcome headaches and stomach upsets. BODs rescues me when I am anxious, especially before speaking engagements.

In my psychotherapy practice, BODs is most helpful between sessions and occasionally during sessions. BODs relaxes me, clears up my mind, and helps me focus. When I am working with a client, my outbreath emanates not from the mouth with pursed lips but from the nose and throat area. This type of breathing — in yoga it is called *ujjai* breathing — enables me to use BODs without intruding on the situation.

Dick Kellor
Retired scientist,
cross-country skier

I participated in Betsy's BreatheOutDynamic system special-interest session at the 2009 Ski for Light event near Provo, Utah, with about thirty other Nordic (cross-country) skiers, both sighted and blind. After hearing Betsy explain BODs, I found myself having to relearn how to breathe. And, the more I practiced BODs, the easier it got. When climbing those ski hills at Soldier Hollow (the 2002 Olympic cross-country ski venue), I used BODs and found it really helped my endurance and adjustment to higher elevations (5,000 to 7,000 feet above sea level). Probably because of dehydration, I experienced several bronchial spasms during the ski outing, and again BODs helped me through these difficult situations.

Back home, I've used BODs as a sleep aid. I am a chronic insomniac, and focusing my mind and body on BODs has been helpful in getting to sleep.

Alma Alvarez
Student of life

I am a forty-two-year-old realist. I believe you must have spiritual strength to help you go through life. My physical strength is limited because I was born with muscular dystrophy. I use a wheelchair for mobility and have limited use of my hands. This is a reality from which I cannot hide. I learned to accept this a long time ago.

In 2004, Betsy Thomason became my respiratory therapist, making monthly home visits to check my breathing machines. For sleep, I use a ventilator with a nasal mask that breathes for me. I use a cough machine a few times a day to stretch my lungs and breathing muscles and to move normal secretions around. In addition, Betsy introduced me to the BreatheOutDynamic system.

Learning and using BODs has helped me relieve anxiety — like my heart is going to leap out of my chest — menstrual cramps, and tightness when I move my bowels. Now that I know how beneficial BODs really is, I practice at least twice a day. BODs reinforces positive thinking and feelings about myself. My mind and body go to a quiet place.

Elaine Hinsch
Skier, sailor, risk taker

I developed asthmatic bronchitis ten years ago when my husband died after a long illness. Being his primary caregiver took its toll on my health. For many years afterward, I was in denial about the severity of my health problem. I would be admitted to the hospital once or twice a year for seven to ten days. One time a doctor told me that if I had waited twenty minutes longer to get to the ER, I would have been intubated and placed on a breathing machine.

In 2008, I decided that I wanted to go on an around-the-world trip visiting old historic sites like Machu Picchu, Easter Island, and Tibet, and so I signed up for a twenty-three-day trip. I brought all my meds with me. My roommate was my friend, who is also my health care proxy. She has seen me through some tough times. When we got to Africa after being in China, where the air quality was very poor, I began to have respiratory symptoms. My roommate wanted me to fly home, but I kept saying, "One more day, just one more day." The trip doctor reassured me that I was making progress. The one thing I was doing differently was using the BreatheOutDynamic system *all* the time. I could feel BODs helping to loosen all the secretions in my airway. Thanks to BODs I was able to stay focused on helping my body recover.

Upon returning home after twenty-three days, I had a chest X-ray. While I had wheezes, I did not have pneumonia or any fluid in my lungs, as I usually would. This was the first time in ten years that I did not have to be hospitalized. Thank you, BODs.

It has been almost two years since I've been hospitalized. I feel stronger than ever. BODs continues to help me overcome my respiratory limitations. Now I'm walking on a treadmill and applying my BODs knowledge to expand my experiences and abilities.

SALIHOU DJABI (1945–2015)
Imam, community activist,
prison chaplain

I was born in the Republic of Guinea, West Africa, and came to America as an adult in 1972. For the past twenty years, I have been the administrative chaplain at Rikers Island prison in New York City. In addition, I am imam of Imam Ali Mosque in Brooklyn, NY, and president of the African Imam Council, Inc., a fellowship of twenty-eight New York mosques.

In 2009, I was diagnosed with ALS (Lou Gehrig's disease), a crippling deadly illness that puts a grown man back into the baby cradle. When I first attended the ALS Clinic at Mount Sinai Beth Israel in New York City, where I met Betsy Thomason, I rode my bike from Brooklyn. By 2011, I was having difficulty using my hands and even walking ten blocks, so I used the BreatheOutDynamic system with every step.

The last thing ALS does is to squeeze your breath out of you, and that is the end of life. To all who are suffering from ALS, do not despair. Allah (God) said: "For every illness there is a cure." Humans have to look for the cure, which is in the universe.

The BreatheOutDynamic system helps patients like me breathe well and effectively. I can feel that breathing from the diaphragm the BODs way is energizing my whole body. Life is breath, and BODs is the most effective way to breathe.

[Editor's note: Imam Djabi died in 2015 from respiratory failure related to ALS.]

ANTHONY NELSON
Athlete, adventurer, single parent,
community leader

Since 1975, I have been involved in all kinds of sports, starting with track and field and wrestling in high school, and more recently cross-country skiing and cycling. In 1988 I represented the United States in the Paralympics in Seoul, Korea, in track and field in the 1500 meters.

My first experience playing with my breathing—really my outbreath—was when I was preparing for the Paralympics tryouts. I was determined to be on the team. I knew my running and jumping skills needed improving—I could not break a five-minute mile, had trouble breathing, and lost energy near the finish. I decided to research the problem and take action. That's when I started paying attention to my breathing. I played with how many strides I was taking for an outbreath and how many for an inbreath. I had no idea I was using the BreatheOutDynamic system. Remarkable things began to happen. I was running faster and longer without panting at the end of a run or race. I cracked the five-minute mile and began running sub-five-minute miles consistently. I started sharing my findings with others. Then I went to Seoul!

In 2009, at Ski for Light, a program that connects sighted skiers with blind people like me, I met Betsy Thomason, RRT, who introduced us skiers to the BreatheOutDynamic system. She immediately got my attention. I explained how I had been using and sharing my own insights about the outbreath.

As a new cross-country skier, I was able to use BODs immediately because I was familiar with the active outbreath. This helped me enjoy gliding up and zooming down the hills at Soldier Hollow near Provo, Utah. Now, when I'm home in South Carolina, I use BODs when walking or cycling, and for relaxation and stress management.

I know that no matter how your health is or what activities you may be involved in, BODs practice will make a big difference in your life, as it has in mine. 🌀

GORDON LARSON
Retired ophthalmologist,
lover of the outdoors
and self-propelled activities

In the early 1950s I discovered the marvels of progressive weight training. By incrementally increasing my efforts I could expand my abilities to bike, hike, and run. At that time, I was focusing on how much air I could take in. To me "belly breathing" meant forcing the belly out on the inhale. Only later in life did I realize that proper breathing enhances these pursuits.

In 2010, I attended Betsy Thomason's BreatheOutDynamic system lecture, an après-ski event at Ski for Light, and that's when I gained understanding of the active outbreath.

But that's only half of my BODs story. It wasn't until the 2011 Ski for Light at Snow Mountain Ranch, 8,750 feet above sea level in the Colorado Rockies, that I grasped the significance of the passive, relaxed inbreath. For most of us lowlanders, just climbing stairs at this high altitude is noticeably harder because the air has 26% less oxygen than at sea level. Now consider that we are cross-country skiing most of the daylight hours!

Here's what Betsy says: practice and focus on the exhale part of breathing. Forget the inhale part—it will take care of itself. So this experienced lowlander did just that. While climbing a steep hill to the dining hall, I invited another skier to focus on what Betsy had just demonstrated. "BODs is very simple," she had said. And indeed it was. We focused on the active outbreath and breezed right up that hill with no breathlessness—proving the presence, and the power, of the passive inbreath.

Amazing—a chance to immediately practice at high altitude. And we passed muster. No need to wearily trudge up that hill—even after a full day of Nordic skiing.

For the rest of the week, David Furukawa, my first-time blind skier, and I practiced BODs, as Betsy had instructed. On the sixth day, during the three-mile race/rally, there was a driving sleet and snowstorm. The twenty-mile-an-hour wind obliterated most of the ski tracks, increasing the effort needed to move forward. We focused on our outbreath, and laughed and cried our way to the finish line.

Betsy's passion for BODs helped David relax and learn to ski in jig time. David and I continue to support each other in our BODs practice and look forward to sharing it with our future skiing companions.

Now, it's your turn to use the BreatheOutDynamic system to fine-tune your life.

REALITY CHECK
EXPANDING YOUR BODs PRACTICE

1. What are your BODs discoveries?
2. What do you dream of being and doing?
3. How are you applying BODs in your life?

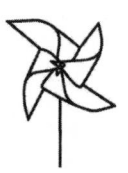

CHAPTER 2

BUILDING THE CASE FOR
THE BREATHEOUTDYNAMIC
SYSTEM
PROOF IS IN YOUR BODY

> "You can't argue with success."
> *Ian Jackson,*
> *outbreath master*

I was walking in my suburban neighborhood with my friend Ellen Hayes, an environmental community organizer with a background in immunochemistry. We were filling in the blanks since our last visit. The BreatheOutDynamic system always claims a big chunk of our conversation.

"So," I said, "here's my challenge: I'm changing the world one person, one breath at a time. Most doctors want a large-scale scientific research study to prove that BODs creates a beneficial outcome in their particular specialty."

We were both quiet for a while, walking and focusing on BODs. Then Ellen set my mind at ease, saying,

"Observation is the first step in the scientific method."

"Thank you, Ellen, for reminding me!"

OBSERVATION AND PERSONAL EXPERIENCE

My passion for the BreatheOutDynamic system led me to enroll in Bergen Community College in 1990 to earn an associate degree in respiratory therapy. My goal was to be a better breathing trainer. Initially, I did not understand the nature of my educational commitment: first, I had to *become* a respiratory therapist.

The course of study was very demanding, even stressful. Besides the academic subjects, there was clinical training — learning how to care for critically ill people with life-threatening breathing problems. Using BODs for relaxation and concentration, I was able to manage stress and overcome my insecurities. After graduation, I passed two national exams to become a registered respiratory therapist (RRT) and became licensed to practice in New Jersey. Then I started a self-prescribed two-year internship in a hospital Intensive Care Unit (ICU) to *really become* a respiratory therapist. I did not know exactly what was in store for me, only that I needed to experience being an ICU-based respiratory therapist.

My ICU assignment was the most challenging work I had ever encountered. During a twelve-hour shift, I was managing a half-dozen or so patients who were intubated (connected to an artificial airway) and hooked up to a mechanical ventilator. Most often they were comatose from overwhelming dysfunction of their lungs, as well as dysfunctions of interrelated organs such as the heart, kidneys, and brain stem. I drew blood directly from arteries or indwelling catheters (flexible tube) to measure levels of oxygen, carbon dioxide, and pH (numerical scale representing acidity or alkalinity of a solution), all of which are affected by breathing, whether mechanical or actual. Sometimes I worked in the emergency room where clear-headed thinking and evaluation were required in view of gross swelling, massive bleeding, or blue pallor.

As always, I used my BODs skills for my own peace of mind. Then I discovered new ways of using BODs I had never even imagined and began to realize that the needs of my patients often fell outside the traditional respiratory therapy protocols.

I remember the time when I was assigned a newly intubated ICU patient. She was awake and alert, but looked frightened to death and was breathing rapidly, despite being on a ventilator. She was connected to a monitor that measured all her vital signs via catheters laced through her arteries into her heart. I made eye contact with her and asked her to use her imagination and pretend she was blowing up a balloon. She played along with me. As I watched the monitor, I saw her blood pressure and her respiratory rate normalize. Then she let the ventilator trigger all her breaths—a good thing—so she would not have to work so hard. Her blood oxygen saturation (referred to as SpO_2) improved. All these measurements demonstrated the power of the BreatheOutDynamic system. Years later, I learned that what I was actually observing was her autonomic nervous system bringing itself back into balance.

After that, as time permitted, I began to teach basic BODs to my ICU patients. I had learned from Ian Jackson, BODs founder, to teach it through metaphors, like the bellows, pinwheel, or balloon. Jackson always said, "Muscles learn best with a mental picture of the task."

Then my supervisor asked me to teach BODs to a longtime smoker who had been intubated on a ventilator for many months and had failed several attempts to breathe on his own. He admitted being afraid that he would not know how to breathe when the tube was removed from his airway (extubation). When my patient assignments allowed, I would guide him through BODs instruction. After a few weeks of using BODs while intubated, he finally went home breathing on his own— no ventilator needed.

So, I thought, this is what it means to *become* a respiratory therapist.

BODs Research

The first BODs (then called BreathPlay) research was conducted at the University of Toledo in 1985. Because BODs was designed by an athlete who trained other athletes, particularly cyclists, this study examined how BODs influenced the performance of twenty-five world-class cyclists. The researchers presented their findings as a poster at the 1987 annual meeting of the American College of Sports Medicine.

In 1989, I conducted the only other BODs study. I wanted to observe how learning and using BODs would affect firefighters' use of self-contained breathing apparatus (SCBA). A small group of Newark, New Jersey, firefighters participated. I presented my research findings as a poster at the 2011 annual meeting of the American College of Chest Physicians.

Both studies are detailed below.

BODs Study with World-Class Cyclists

The 1985 University of Toledo study was conducted by exercise physiologists Daniel M. Wojta and Xavier F. Flores (also a respiratory therapist), while earning doctorate and master's degrees, respectively. Their purpose was to compare the before and after performance of two groups

of elite athletes. The experimental group, fifteen members
of the Maumee Valley Wheelmen, a member club of the
United States Cycling Federation (USCF), spent three days
with Ian Jackson learning BODs. The control group, ten
top USCF triathletes from northwestern Ohio, received
no BODs training. Both groups were tested for endurance
before the experimental group received BODs training.
Two to three weeks later, both groups were retested.

Results of the University of Toledo BODs
study were statistically significant, as reported by the
University of Toledo Office of Public Information in a
March 31, 1987, press release, and on April 6, 1987, in the
Collegian, the University of Toledo student newspaper.
In the experimental group, endurance was increased by
7.2%. This translates into the experimental group being
able to pedal two minutes farther — before becoming
exhausted — than the cyclists who did not learn BODs. In
scientific terms, exhaustion is defined as the point where
the body switches its main source of energy from fats
burned in the presence of oxygen to energy derived from
burning stored carbohydrates without oxygen. Practically
speaking, exhaustion occurs when huffing and puffing
starts and muscles become heavy — evidence of lactic acid
buildup. For world-class cyclists, two minutes is a huge
edge when racing. In addition, the perceived exertion
reported by the experimental group was reduced by 9.6%.

How did the researchers explain the gain of the
BODs cyclists?

In the 1987 press release, Mr. Wojta said, "The mechanism is still uncertain, but our evidence points to more efficient breathing among experimental subjects as compared to the control group, as seen in lowered heart rates, decreased perceived exertion, and greater endurance."

In the same press release, Mr. Flores noted that using BODs, "forceful expiration appears to produce a rebound effect, which may be responsible for a more effortless inspiration."

In an April 13, 2001, email to me, Ian Jackson explained his understanding of the results this way: "The researchers at the University of Toledo pointed out to me that the muscle work of normal breathing (with healthy lungs and respiratory muscles) costs about 10% of oxygen uptake, leaving 90% for the work of riding. They believed that the BODs riders' ability to pedal longer than the control group of cyclists indicated a dramatic reduction in the oxygen-cost of breathing" — also called reduced work of breathing. In the long run, whether you have a breathing problem and use an arm bike for exercise or you are a world-class cyclist powering over the Pyrenees, BODs proof is in *your* pedals.

BODs Study with Newark, New Jersey, Firefighters

In 1988, I was pondering who specifically would benefit from learning BODs. I already knew that cyclists and hikers would be interested in decreased huffing and puffing. But one day, while brainstorming with several volunteer firefighter friends, it dawned on me that they knew lots of folks who were always "close" to their breathing. This sparked an idea for training and research.

The purpose of my research was to discover how the use of BODs would affect firefighters' air consumption during physical exertion. I wanted to determine if firefighters who use BODs could extend the length of time their self-contained breathing apparatus (SCBA) would last. I hypothesized that, with BODs passive, relaxed inbreath, there would be slower depletion of air in the tank on the firefighter's back.

In March 1989, seven hazmat (hazardous materials) firefighters from Truck 1 in the Newark, New Jersey, Fire Department signed on to the research project. They took a pretest and began BODs training. The pretest established the number of laps of a walking course each participant could complete before their SCBA emptied. Because of the demands of their workplace, just three of the original seven firefighters completed BODs instruction. Following the fourth training session, Paul, Chuck, and Billy (their names have been changed) repeated the pretest. The average number of laps completed before the SCBA ran out of air increased by an amazing 32%. Paul expanded his abilities from 11½ laps to 17 laps; Chuck from 10 to 14 laps; and Billie from 10 to 11 laps.

Paul, a smoker for fourteen years who walked every

day for an hour or two, said that BODs allowed him to control his breathing rate and was useful for regimented exercise.

Chuck, a former smoker who did not exercise regularly, stated, "Despite having smoked and not exercising, I discovered that with BODs I can increase my breathing efficiency just by breathing upside down (focusing on the outbreath)."

Billie had smoked for thirty-five years, did not exercise, and complained of a hiatal hernia, a painful condition where stomach tissue is squeezed by the diaphragm. He evaluated his experience this way: "BODs showed me a new method of conserving air in my SCBA and how to relax under stressful situations. I learned that I can help myself physically by letting my brain and body work together."

VALIDATION

People have been breathing for a long time by natural design, with great benefit. Is it necessary to authenticate BODs with evidence-based research? Or can we rely on our own observations combined with age-old scientific knowledge? You be the judge. Several basic physics principles explain how air enters the human body. BODs methodology utilizes all these understandings.

FIRST PHYSICS PRINCIPLE: The duo of *vacuum and suction* work together—first to push fluid or gas out of a space, then to let fluid or gas flow into the space, respectively. In Italy in 1643, Evangelista Torricelli created and documented the first laboratory vacuum. So whether the container is a bellows or your lungs, vacuum and suction harmoniously empty, then fill, the space because of a change in pressure. During BODs active, spine-stretching outbreath, contents of the abdomen push up against the diaphragm, forcing air out, creating higher pressure inside the chest than outside — vacuum. Out goes the air. When the abdominal muscles are released with BODs passive, relaxed inbreath, the chest space expands naturally, creating higher pressure outside the body than inside — suction. In comes air without physical effort.

SECOND PHYSICS PRINCIPLE: *Gravity* claims that everything is attracted to everything else based on mass. Sir Isaac Newton published his Law of Universal Gravitation in 1687. In the twentieth century, Albert Einstein restated this as his Theory of General Relativity. Typically, we think of gravity as a pulling toward the center of the earth. This is due to the planet's mass. When you are focusing on BODs while standing or sitting, gravity helps move your diaphragm toward the floor — and thus the center of the earth — just enough to expand your lungs downward about an inch. When you are lying flat, your diaphragm no longer moves toward the floor, so gravity cannot help. This explains why breathing is shallow during sleep on a flat bed. It's okay, as long as your respiratory muscles are strong and your airway is not obstructed.

THIRD PHYSICS PRINCIPLE: *Recoil* states that for every action there is an equal and opposite reaction. Sir Isaac Newton published this in 1687 as his third Law of Motion. Recoil describes the action at the end of BODs active, spine-stretching outbreath when abdominal muscles are released, instantly providing space for the diaphragm's descent. This recoil invites air into the lungs effortlessly — BODs innate feature. Most other breathing practices focus on an active inbreath, which wastes precious energy.

BODs collaborates with vacuum/suction, gravity, and recoil to reduce the work of breathing for everyone. Thus, centuries-old scientific theories — long ago considered fact — support the logic of BODs active, spine-stretching outbreath and its passive, relaxed inbreath.

More BODs validation comes gratis from the American Heart Association (AHA). In 2010, the AHA changed its decades-old procedure for cardiopulmonary resuscitation (CPR), first aid for people assessed to be in the midst of a heart attack. The new AHA protocol, called "hands-only CPR," eliminates mouth-to-mouth breathing. Now, CPR starts with 30 chest compressions at a rate of 100 per minute, pushing to a depth of 2 inches. This hard, fast action creates increased pressure inside the chest cavity, massaging the heart, moving blood around, and stimulating the return of heartbeat and blood flow. This downward action of chest compressions also influences the lungs, pushing air out—outbreath. In between split-second compressions, pressure in the chest cavity decreases, creating a vacuum. With this pressure change, air rushes into the lungs—inbreath—with no need for mouth-to-mouth resuscitation.

This new CPR protocol exactly defines the BreatheOutDynamic system: active spine-stretching outbreath—CPR chest compression—and passive, relaxed inbreath—that instant between each chest compression when air enters. Philadelphia cardiologist Ramesh Adiraju, MD, confirms this: "The chest-compressions-only CPR protocol is equivalent to BODs." Thank you, American Heart Association, for your change in protocol, which validates BODs.

If BODs works in an emergency, it should work all the time. But you have to practice BODs to incorporate it into your muscle memory. So let's get started. Your own experiences will keep you moving forward on your path through life. Then you can tell your own personal BODs story.

REALITY CHECK
BEGINNING YOUR BODs PRACTICE

1. What BODs concepts intrigue you?

2. What is your commitment to your BODy?

3. How might BODs benefit your well-being?

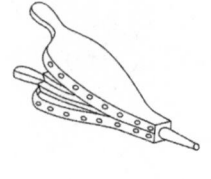

THE BODS BASICS

CHAPTER 3

LEARN THE BREATHEOUTDYNAMIC SYSTEM

THE TWO-STEP BASICS

"Nothing works unless you do."
Maya Angelou,
American author

"When you're finished changing, you're finished."
Fortune cookie wisdom

Every human being lives from one breath to the next. If you don't breathe, you are not living. If you hold your breath, you are not living well. If you never pay attention to your breathing, you are missing the many benefits of effective breathing.

Kevin Trotta, a bicyclist who lives in the Hudson Highlands sixty miles north of New York City, knows full well the importance of breathing. For years he's been pedaling twenty to thirty miles several times per week along the mountainous roads that cling to the side of Storm King Mountain whose steep cliffs touch the Hudson River. He has always used breath to fuel his rides. But it wasn't until Kevin met up with Lou Gehrig's disease (amyotrophic lateral sclerosis, or ALS) that he discovered the power of the outbreath. "When my doctor introduced me to the ALS Team respiratory therapist, Betsy Thomason, she helped me manage stress with BODs. Neither of us realized its full potential for me." Kevin continues to ride even though his left leg is weak. How does he manage? He powers the left pedal with his outbreath, and courage. "BODs is what's keeping me riding," he says with a twinkle in his eye. "You can't see my limp when I'm riding!"

The primary purpose of breathing is to manage the energy required by each cell in the human body. In our modern, revved-up culture, we humans live on autopilot. This works for machines but is not effective for the human body. As a result, breathing, which is both an automatic process and a conscious, focused process, is sorely neglected, and its significance is lost. Brains are running the automatic show. Bodies are simply dragged along for the ride, often bumpy at best. However, bodies always have the last word, like it or not.

REDEFINING BREATHING

BODs is inherently fun and creative and best understood through the use of metaphors. Thus, BODs incorporates images like blowing on a pinwheel and squeezing a fireplace bellows to explain the *out-in* breathing process and enhance learning. Ultimately, BODs helps you access your core muscles — the abdominals, your bellows. This girdle of muscles between your hips, from the arch of your lower ribs to your pelvic bone, is called your "core" because it supports your entire body. It is your energy center. When you use your abdominals to generate a long outbreath, you are not only breathing efficiently, you are exercising your abdominal muscles and protecting your low back at the same time. Indeed, you are influencing every muscle and every organ in your body because the core is like a crossroads. Everything is connected to everything. All systems require well-oxygenated blood for full, pain-free functioning. In this entire breathing-out process, you are getting acquainted with your body. Once you start to use your belly muscles to accompany the long outbreath, you start to experience a calm that brings relaxation and self-awareness.

The BreatheOutDynamic system is focused breathing with emphasis on the *active, spine-stretching outbreath and passive, relaxed inbreath*. This cycle of outbreath and inbreath is just the opposite of what is considered "normal" breathing. BODs challenges the age-old assumption that breathing is an in-out process. The BODs *out-in* focus is based on ancient esoteric wisdom from yoga and martial-arts masters. By using this out-in orientation, BODs users efficiently expand their physical and mental abilities.

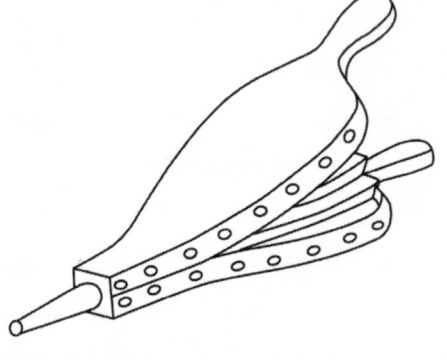

3.1

The bellows metaphor explains the efficiency of the
BreatheOutDynamic system.

The BreatheOutDynamic system teaches you a new way to look at life—*at your life*—the only one you can change. You will learn a new way of releasing carbon dioxide into your surrounding environment and *allowing* life-giving oxygen to enter your internal environment without effort. This give-and-take is the simplicity of BODs, which can make a real difference in your life.

Over the years, I have used the bellows as one of the metaphors for the BreatheOutDynamic system. I encourage my students to "be the bellows!" When you squeeze something, then suddenly expand it, you create a vacuum followed by suction—a universal law of physics. The bellows image suggests that if you push the air out of your body using your belly—creating the vacuum— assisted by gently pursed lips, the same amount of air comes bounding back automatically, and fast, the instant your belly expands—creating suction. So try this long, active, spine-stretching outbreath, followed by a brief, passive, and relaxed inbreath. Voila. An effective breath with half the effort. This is basic BODs.

When you practice BODs and get in touch with your body rhythms and messages and trust that nature's vacuum works, you will experience the rich complexity of the BreatheOutDynamic system.

BODs Basic Two-Step

Outbreath
BODs Step #1
Simultaneously squeeze your belly muscles—close the bellows—and blow out gently through pursed lips. These actions push air out of your lungs and slow down the flow of air out through your mouth.

Inbreath
BODs Step #2
Now simultaneously release your belly muscles—open the bellows—and stop blowing out, *allowing* the universe

to refill your lungs. Your only task is to *let* your belly muscles relax. You've just started learning the BreatheOutDynamic system.

PRACTICING BODs
BASIC TWO-STEP

To initially teach your muscles the BreatheOutDynamic system, practice three times a day, for 5 to 15 minutes or more. Find a quiet place with no television, no electronics — no distractions. It might be when you are falling asleep or waking up, and then one other time, sitting in a straight-backed chair, perhaps before a meal. With this quiet BODs practice, you will become deeply acquainted with your body. Experience the ebb and flow — the out and in — of your breath. Notice the action of your spine against the mattress or the back of the chair during the outbreath. Be with your body. Be in praise of your body — that is, be nonjudgmental. Enjoy what you are accomplishing. You are preparing to use BODs with movement, whether getting out of bed or running a marathon.

EXPANDING THE BELLOWS METAPHOR

To gain more understanding of your body, let's examine the bellows metaphor. How does the bellows work? How does air reenter the bellows? How do you know that air has come back into the bellows?

The work of the bellows begins when human hands squeeze the bellows, pushing air out through its narrow opening onto an ember to encourage fire. As soon as human hands reopen the bellows, air enters the narrow opening because of a sudden change in internal pressure. While you can't actually see air enter, you can observe that the bellows has expanded. Observation is the first step in understanding natural phenomena. Observing that you can squeeze the bellows again and again and experience the same gush of air out confirms this physics principle.

Admittedly, the bellows is an imperfect BODs metaphor because the lungs are separate from the belly, and the energy required to refill the lungs is passive recoil — not active recoil as it is with the bellows. However, the BreatheOutDynamic system utilizes the same change in internal pressure that any container uses — bellows, oven baster, or plastic shampoo bottle — to suck a gas or liquid back in. It's the way the universe works.

The bellows expels air through an opening in a narrow tube. In the human body this action is analogous to pursing your lips — the whistling position — and blowing out gently. The benefit of gently restricting air flow with your lips, teeth, or tongue is to create pressure, which keeps the airway open so you can expel more used air. There are additional ways to create restriction without effort. You can blow out against smiling lips or grunt, sing, hum, or whistle.

The bellows metaphor defines the BreatheOutDynamic system in another way. The job of the bellows is to make a fire burn more brightly because air aids combustion. This is accomplished by pushing air out of the bellows onto the embers. Entrance of air back into the bellows, while essential, does not support the fire. This is also true in your body where metabolism is the fire, and your belly is the bellows. The metaphor continues with the breathing cycle of outbreath—squeezing the bellows; and inbreath—expanding the bellows. The outbreath generates power and relaxation while the inbreath simply fills the lungs with air.

Without adequate exchange of carbon dioxide and oxygen, metabolism is sluggish. The body screams for help with messages such as shortness of breath, cramps, heavy legs, chest pressure, brain fog, and anxiety.

Over the years, my students have never questioned that the bellows itself always fills quickly with air. But often I see my students waiting more than three seconds, thinking that air has not yet entered their lungs, or I see them actively sucking in air. They are demonstrating that while their brain understands the bellows' message, their body does not. This is an example of the brain-body disconnect. Does this describe you? Here's a way to observe what really happens.

When practicing the BreatheOutDynamic system, vary the length of time you wait passively for the air to enter your lungs. Using "one, one thousand" to represent one second, count in your head to "four, one thousand" before blowing out again. Do this for a few breaths. Then do the same as you wait for three seconds — or three, one thousand — and so forth, until you finally wait for just one second — one, one thousand. Have you always had air to blow out again, no matter how long you waited? Yes, of course, because nature's vacuum instantly creates suction — without effort — drawing in as much air as was blown out.

You decide how long to wait before blowing out again. The longer you wait, the more likely your body is to take a shallow, inefficient, ineffective breath or two — your old, unconscious breathing habit. Play around with how long to wait for air to reenter your body — one or two seconds should suffice. It all depends upon what you are doing or experiencing.

Learning and applying a new idea, one that turns your world upside down, is a challenge. It is easier to learn something brand new than to change an old habit like in-out breathing. This is why I recommend that you forget about undoing "normal" in-out breathing. Just become committed to the BreatheOutDynamic system. Simply add it to your daily routine and trust BODs to connect you with all the energy you need.

THE IRONIC POWER OF THE PASSIVE, RELAXED INBREATH

Consider this: one outstanding feature of the BreatheOutDynamic system is its passive, relaxed inbreath—just the opposite of "regular" breathing. The irony is that most active, high-functioning people avoid being passive. The BODs inbreath is one instance in life when passivity is to your advantage. During the BODs passive inbreath, the diaphragm, the most important muscle of respiration, is expending little energy to do its hardest work—expanding the lungs downward. This represents a net gain of energy for your entire body.

PHYSICAL EDUCATION AND PRACTICE

Becoming committed to the BreatheOutDynamic system is not difficult. But it does require time for practice, because this is physical education, not intellectual brain training.

"Education of the physical body is a huge and important undertaking, and should not be left to chance," says Lee Coleman, MA, professor emeritus of physical education at Whitman College in Walla Walla, Washington. "The goals of physical education are much broader than simply training for success in sports, athletics, and recreation. Physical education should emphasize rhythm, repetition, and relaxation. At its best, physical education enriches and sustains all aspects of life. Infants and toddlers learn largely through their physical movement—trial and error leading to understanding. In an ideal environment, young children should have endless movement opportunities with minimal hours logged on TV, video games, and the latest technological device. Children who enter school fit and who love to use their bodies are a physical educator's dream and a classroom teacher's joy. Such physical education needs to be applied throughout one's lifetime, not just during childhood.

"The starting point for effective movement is efficient breathing. Everyone can breathe, but few have learned—then practiced—good technique. Practice is necessary to master any motor skill. But practice must be of the perfect technique to be worthwhile. The BreatheOutDynamic system is perfect technique," Coleman says.

You are teaching your muscles a new approach to breathing. Different kinds of muscles have different jobs. When given a chance, each muscle knows how to perform its own job. But muscles like the abdominals that have been neglected, as in a beer belly, or overused, as in military posture—guts *always* sucked in—forget how to behave. So muscles need your conscious help to do their best. They are smart but require practice and a nonjudgmental brain in order to develop their craft.

USING YOUR IMAGINATION

Muscles respond to pictures of what you want them to do. But not everyone responds to the same image or metaphor. So, *you* can develop a metaphor consistent with your own understanding of BODs, human body design, and your life experiences. One caution: blowing out a candle is not a valid image because the outbreath knocks the flame off the wick, extinguishing the candle. The BODs outbreath *increases* the internal flame, your metabolism.

Here's another BODs metaphor: the belly-button string. Think of your belly button as a real button with two holes in it. Now lace a string into the holes and bring the string straight back through your spine. Pretend to grab the string and pull the button back toward your spine to accomplish the outbreath. Release the string to initiate the inbreath.

Feel free to expand upon these metaphors or create your own. One of my students suggested that if you physically pull the imaginary string, it becomes an exercise for the triceps muscle located on the back of the upper arm. She recommended alternating arms so both arms benefit.

Be-a-Balloon is another BODs game you can play. It is an exception to the concept of the passive, relaxed inbreath and is meant for stationary exercise only. But it is important because chest wall muscles like to be stretched, and BODs passive inbreath, though efficient, does not stretch muscles very much.

Try this: pretend that your belly and chest are a pear-shaped balloon. While sitting or lying down, do a few BODs cycles of active, spine-stretching outbreath and passive, relaxed inbreath. Then, after an active outbreath, release your belly quickly and feel it expand, then let that energy-wave glide into your chest. Feel the expansion of your chest, the top part of the imaginary pear-shaped balloon. When you feel the wave reach your throat, bring your belly button toward your spine to deflate the balloon, then refill the balloon a few times. Each active outbreath *and* active inbreath might take 6 to 10 seconds or more — really slow and exaggerated.

Consider Be-a-Balloon a BODs yawn. It stretches both the chest wall and the lung tissue. It's okay to put extra effort into the Be-a-Balloon inbreath when you are stationary because you are not using energy to move your limbs.

If you play Be-a-Balloon lying flat, notice that your shoulders are stationary. This is helpful because lungs are not attached to shoulders, but rather to the diaphragm. When we sit or stand and take a traditional deep inbreath, we habitually raise our shoulders—without benefit. The BreatheOutDynamic system eliminates this wasteful movement.

I credit Be-a-Balloon with solving my lifelong ticklish-rib problem. Every time a friend or family member put an arm around my waist, I would jump. This did not seem normal to me. Knowing that muscles that are not moved often become twitchy, mine included, I did a BODs experiment. I did daily Be-a-Balloon repetitions. After regular practice for a month or so, my tickle problem disappeared. Now I no longer jump at the flick of an arm around my waist.

Another BODs metaphor is the pinwheel, which spins only when you blow on it. An amazing thing happens whether you are blowing on a real or imagined pinwheel. Your belly automatically tightens and moves toward your spine—outbreath. In the instant that you stop blowing, your belly relaxes outward—inbreath. This unconscious movement is exactly what you consciously focus on when doing BODs. Your pinwheel is virtually always with you.

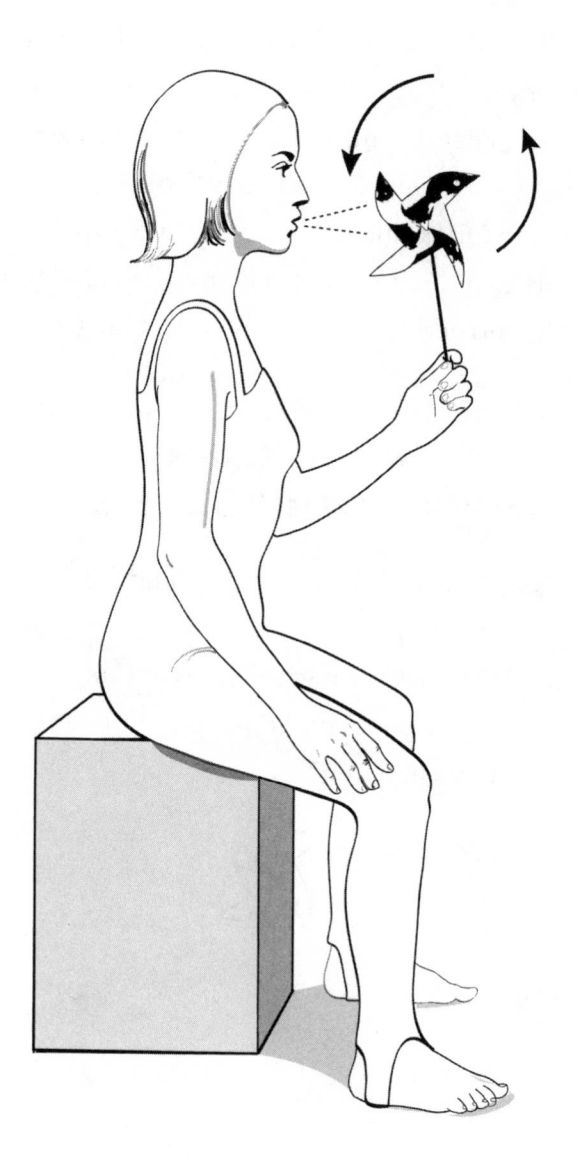

3.2

*The pinwheel metaphor reminds us that we are powered
by our outbreath.*

Over the years, I have had fun teaching people how to practice BODs by turning the pinwheel metaphor into reality. First, we make pinwheels, then we play with them. Bingo! Students immediately see the power of their outbreath and the value of pursed lips and passive inbreath. This leads to a discussion of how to apply BODs in daily life. At the end of this book, you'll find a pinwheel template and directions for making your very own pinwheel.

REALITY CHECK
EXPANDING YOUR BODs PRACTICE

1. What is your new understanding of breathing?
2. Which BODs metaphors work for you?
3. How is your relationship with your body changing?

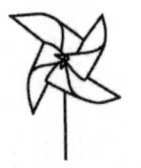

CHAPTER 4

HOW YOUR BODY WORKS

RETHINKING BREATHING

> "If you learn only methods you'll be tied to your
> methods, but if you learn principles you
> can devise your own methods."
> *Ralph Waldo Emerson,*
> *American philosopher*

The human body is thoughtfully designed. Air, the most important substance for human existence, enters your body automatically, freely, and without thought. That is the way the universe works. What a gift.

However, this gift of unconscious breathing has its downside. Lack of attention creates a failure to understand the expansiveness of breathing. The actions used to exchange gases within the human body can also create a range of experiences — everything from relaxation to distress, and strength to weakness. If you are not paying attention to your breathing, you are not paying attention to the wide range of accompanying physical and emotional responses. You are not using the primary life-management tool that is available to everyone at all times — breathing.

How is the body designed to integrate breathing with so many body and mind functions? A look at basic anatomy and physiology of breathing will expand your understanding.

STRUCTURE

A trip along the airway
from nose to alveoli

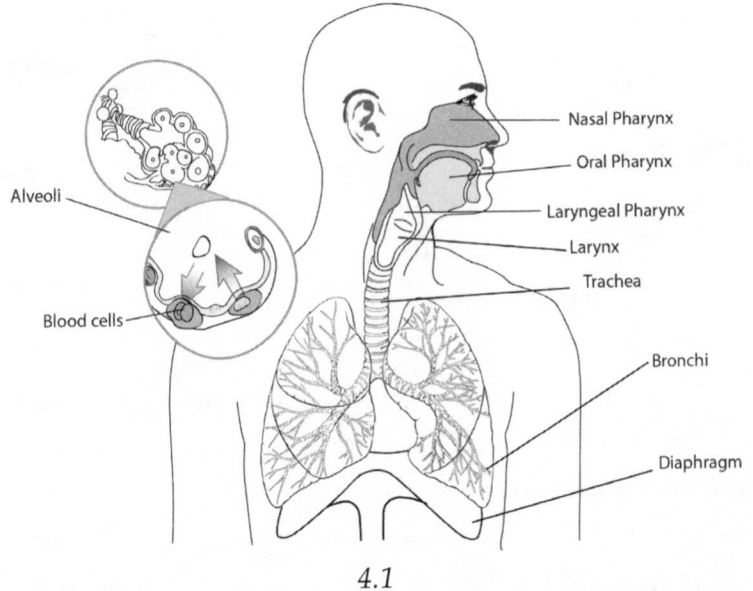

Alveoli

Blood cells

Nasal Pharynx

Oral Pharynx

Laryngeal Pharynx

Larynx

Trachea

Bronchi

Diaphragm

4.1

Basic breathing guideposts from nose to alveoli
and capillaries are described in the text.

The nose, that landmark jutting out of the face, invites air to enter its two hallways, called nares or nostrils, where air is heated, humidified, and filtered. The mouth can also funnel air toward the lungs, especially during fast-paced exercise. One precaution: habitual mouth breathing is not healthy.

THE PERILS OF MOUTH BREATHING

The habit of mouth breathing dries up mucous membranes, an open invitation for nasty microbes to enter the body—through gums, teeth, or any surface of the mouth. Over time, increased air flow pushes the roof of the mouth—the palate—up into the nasal cavities, diminishing their size, causing a cascade of effects. In addition, air can move front teeth forward, creating an open bite that further keeps the mouth open.

There are many causes for mouth breathing. Clogged sinuses are both a cause and effect. To promote healthy sinuses, try cleaning out your sinus cavities by sniffing warm normal saline up your nose every morning. This unclogs nature's filter. Then cough and blow your nose.

Or you can use a neti pot and follow package directions. Normal saline, which is the same salinity as body fluid, can be made using a half teaspoon of pure salt per cup of water.

From the nose, air flows via the nasal pharynx into the throat where it meets the oral pharynx, the back of the throat. The airway continues downward to the laryngeal pharynx, a tubular space into which food and air travel together until they reach the larynx, commonly called the Adam's apple or voice box. The larynx houses vocal cords and connects the laryngeal pharynx to the trachea, commonly called the windpipe. On top of the larynx, a piece of flapping cartilage called the epiglottis closes off the trachea during swallowing to channel food into the esophagus, the tube behind the trachea that leads to the stomach.

To ensure that intruders, like dust or food particles, do not enter the trachea, the body sneezes or coughs. A sneeze, primarily an unconscious process, protects the airway above the larynx. A cough protects the airway below the larynx and can be initiated automatically by sensors in the trachea. A cough can also be generated consciously by taking a big inbreath and exhaling forcefully and fast, against a partially closed glottis, another name for the vocal cords and the space between them. This self-initiated cough is just the opposite of

BODs, for good reason. The movement of lots of air quickly out of your lungs clears your airway of intruders.

To learn more about the next breathing guidepost, touch the "V" in your collarbone directly below the larynx. Now, move your finger down an inch or two and you will feel a speed bump two to three inches wide. This is the top of the sternum, or breastbone, behind which the trachea splits, creating the right bronchus and the left bronchus (two bronchi) — the pathways into the right and left lungs.

The bronchi divide, again and again, becoming narrower and narrower. They simply transport air to the deeper portions of the lungs under the ribs where 300 to 500 million grape-like sacs called alveoli are surrounded by about 3,000 miles of microscopic blood vessels called capillaries. If all goes well in the alveoli, oxygen molecules are sifted out of the air and pass through fluid and a layer of tissue fifty times thinner than onion-skin paper, into the capillaries. (Dean Schraufnagel, MD, editor. *Breathing in America: Diseases, Progress, and Hope.* New York, New York: American Thoracic Society, 2010.)

Then oxygen molecules hop onto hemoglobin (iron molecules in blood) to be pumped by the heart throughout the entire body, feeding hungry cells.

If you are a chest breather or you breathe more than twenty times a minute, air is not getting deep into your lungs where oxygen enters the blood. This may be one of the reasons you might feel chest pressure in the area of the breastbone, because you are stacking one breath on top of another without ever getting rid of old, used air. One possible solution to this problem is learning and using the BreatheOutDynamic system.

The BODs active, spine-stretching outbreath engages the diaphragm, the primary muscle of respiration. This large saucer-shaped muscle that spans the width of the chest cavity right under the ribs is high in the front and low in the back, creating the floor of the lung/heart space and the roof of the abdominal cavity. The rhythmical up-and-down movement of the diaphragm creates small but adequate changes of pressure inside the lungs to expel used air laden with carbon dioxide and then to let in fresh air laden with oxygen. If movement of the diaphragm is impeded by a big belly, weak belly muscles, or a weak diaphragm, the result could be shortness of breath, or your body might just breathe faster to compensate. Faster means shallow and ineffective.

GRASPING HOW THE DIAPHRAGM WORKS TO SAVE ENERGY

To visualize how the diaphragm works, look at your hand. Rest your arm and hand on a table or chair armrest and note the shape of your resting hand. Your fingers are curved, creating a cupped shape. During the BODs active, spine-stretching outbreath, this is the way the diaphragm appears—cupped and *relaxed*. It is ironic that when the diaphragm is working its hardest, helping the human body to be strong, this primary muscle of breathing is at rest! The resulting extraordinary relaxation is why there is no pause between BODs outbreath and inbreath, as there is in regular breathing.

Amazingly, the actual work of the diaphragm occurs during the *inbreath*. To visualize this, stretch your resting fingers. Your hand flattens out. During the inbreath, the diaphragm also flattens out, doing its most important work—pulling lung tissue downward about one inch to expand it. The BODs relaxed inbreath that *lets* air into the lungs because of a change in air pressure requires minimal effort, allowing the diaphragm to work efficiently. Thus, the BreatheOutDynamic system saves energy, reducing the work of breathing during outbreath *and* inbreath.

The two spongy, expandable air compartments we call the right and left lungs are connected to the diaphragm, not the shoulders, so lifting your shoulders to take in a breath is futile. It is an empty gesture. Instead, use your belly like a bellows to squeeze out used air and invite new air in, utilizing the natural elasticity of chest wall muscles and nature's vacuum.

Just getting air into the right location is complex. Now, add the task of removing carbon dioxide, the end product of metabolism. Keep in mind that blood transports carbon dioxide and oxygen simultaneously. Some carbon dioxide must remain in the blood to balance the body's acidity and alkalinity (pH). If you exhale too much carbon dioxide, you will feel light-headed. If you exhale too little carbon dioxide, you will feel tired or drowsy. The happy medium, a state of consistent energy, is achieved by listening to your body.

One of my BODs students was a butcher. He knew more about anatomy than I. He told me that the diaphragm is the body's most highly oxygenated muscle. He said that if you need iron-rich food, eat skirt steak, which is the diaphragm. Even if you don't eat meat, check out skirt steak in the market. Notice how the muscle is constructed. It is flared from the center, like rays of the sun. This design, he said, helps the diaphragm relax and contract with every outbreath and inbreath, respectively.

The secondary muscles of respiration, the intercostals, are located between your ribs. This chest wall mantle of muscle and bone works with the diaphragm, pulling the rib cage down and in, and up and out to alternately squeeze and expand the space. If intercostals are weak or ribs are missing, the unconscious breathing process becomes labored or ineffective.

The back-up breathing strategy, when the diaphragm and chest wall muscles are not fully functional, is to use neck muscles. Try this: gasp for breath. Notice the strain on your neck muscles. They attempt to lift and open your rib cage to force in air. This effort brings in some air but is totally inefficient, creating a huge energy loss, sinking the breather deeper and deeper into oxygen debt. You feel short of breath and wonder how you're going to survive.

You *will* survive because human design includes methods to compensate for loss of the diaphragmatic function. Often though, without awareness, people use rib cage muscles when their diaphragm is potentially fully functional. If you see the top of your shirt moving rhythmically as you breathe, you are *not* engaging your diaphragm. You are not expelling adequate carbon dioxide, and thus CO_2 blocks fresh oxygen-laden air from ever reaching your millions of alveoli. You may feel tired or even sleepy. You may yawn, a giant inbreath. This is your body speaking: "Hello, I'm tired of the same old shallow breaths." The yawn stretches your chest wall to achieve full exchange of air. Your muscles are happier for the duration of the yawn.

Tired of Yawning?

Yawning, traditionally thought to be a sign of intellectual boredom, is a precursor to falling asleep in class, heaven forbid. Actually, yawning is a body message that says that the entire body is bored, tired of the same old, same old — whatever that is. The body, especially muscle, is tired of the routine: sitting at a desk or behind the wheel, or walking mile after level mile. The lungs also get tired from the same small volume of air, breath after breath — not enough oxygen to nourish tissue.

What's the solution? Move your body, change your position, include hills in your walk, and practice the BreatheOutDynamic system to create a happy body.

Now consider the BreatheOutDynamic system. With each outbreath, BODs engages the diaphragm, the primary muscle of respiration. Instead of letting the diaphragm move passively to expel carbon dioxide, the BODs user actively engages the diaphragm by pushing the contents of the belly up against the relaxed — yes, relaxed — diaphragm, forcing it up to squeeze the lungs and thus expel carbon dioxide. Releasing the belly muscles allows the diaphragm to contract and the chest wall muscles to recoil passively to *let* in air, *with little or no effort.*

Why not take advantage of nature's vacuum/ suction and your own innate elastic recoil? This is the vital difference between plain old breathing, other breathing methods, and the BreatheOutDynamic system.

To visualize the difference between plain old breathing and the BreatheOutDynamic system, turn the page. The figures on the left page illustrate the outbreath and inbreath of plain old, normal, unfocused breathing. Read the caption for details.

The figures on the right page illustrate the BreatheOutDynamic system, helping you to see the anatomical differences between BODs outbreath and inbreath. Then, as you compare the differences between normal, unfocused breathing on the left page with the BreatheOutDynamic system on the right page, you gain a deeper understanding of BODs benefits. Read the caption for details.

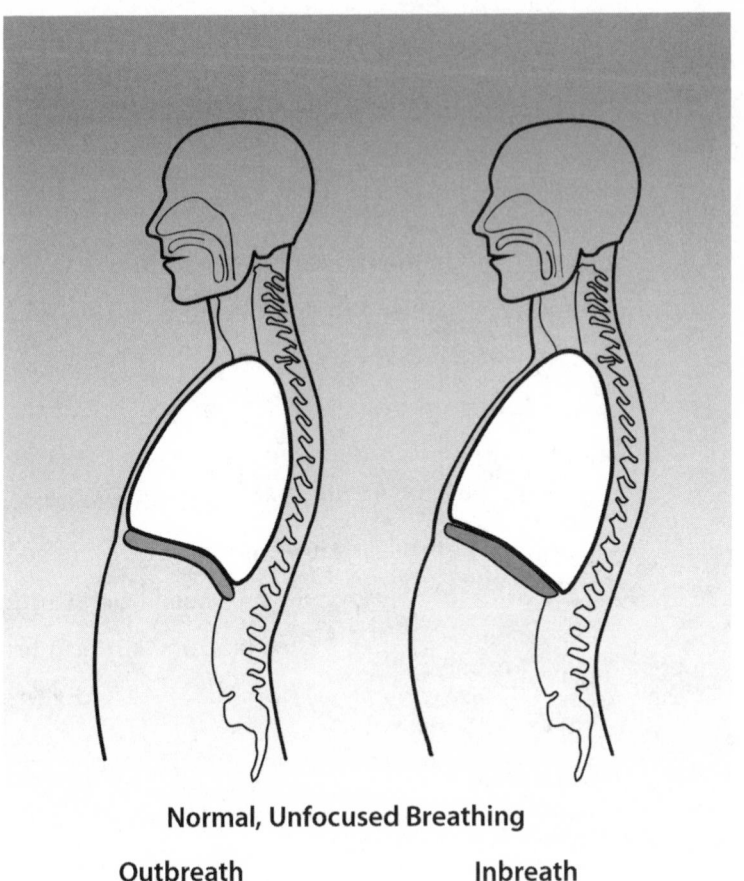

Normal, Unfocused Breathing

Outbreath   **Inbreath**

4.2a

During the "normal" unfocused outbreath (left) and inbreath (right), the belly and diaphragm remain relatively unchanged, essentially not doing their share of the work of breathing. Because of this lack of action, abdominal muscles become weak, providing no stability to the body's core and spine.

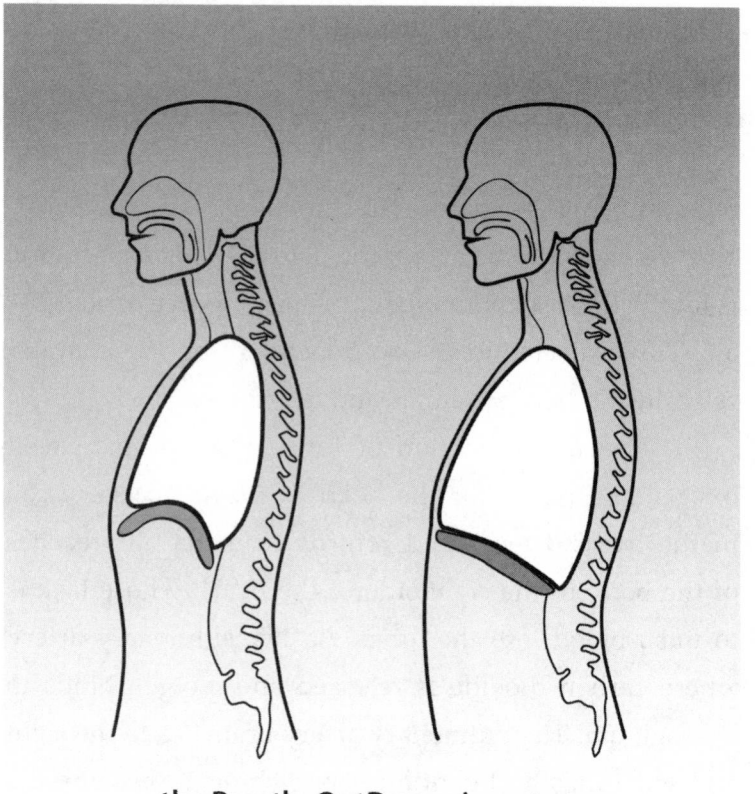

the BreatheOutDynamic system
Outbreath **Inbreath**

4.2b

During BODs outbreath (left) and inbreath (right), the belly and diaphragm dramatically change shape and position to optimize the work of breathing. Because of the outbreath action, abdominal muscles become strong, stabilizing and protecting the body's core and spine. What other changes do you notice?

Function
Enhanced by the use of
the BreatheOutDynamic system

Human beings by nature are functional. We do "stuff," and we expect to be able to do "stuff." This expectation is totally dependent upon our primary source of energy — air. This expectation is also dependent on the complex relationship between lungs and heart. Here's why.

The main function of lungs is to provide well-oxygenated blood for the heart to pump to every cell in the body. Then blood returns from the far reaches of the body to the right side of the heart, whose task is to push blood into the lungs via the pulmonary artery, where carbon dioxide is released and oxygen binds to hemoglobin. The pulmonary artery branches to the right and left lungs and continues branching to become the 3,000-mile network of hairlike capillaries that surround 300 to 500 million alveoli. Carbon dioxide in blood exits through capillary walls into the alveoli. Oxygen does the reverse. Pressure in the system propels oxygenated blood back to the left side of the heart via four pulmonary veins. Refreshed blood pulses through the left side of the heart where pressure builds again to send oxygenated blood on its merry way back to the far reaches of the body.

The way we breathe affects the work of the heart. If you are a chest breather, the little bit of air you take in is mixed with carbon-dioxide-laden air still in your airway. In addition, you are stacking one breath on top of another, never allowing air with 21% oxygen to reach your alveoli. Thus your heart has to beat more often, doing a lot of extra work to push around poorly oxygenated blood.

Unfortunately, in the twenty-first century, the breathing process is ignored, allowed to run on automatic. Our health care is focused on drugs and surgery, not on awareness, personal responsibility, and functional interventions such as the BreatheOutDynamic system.

In his 1986 book *The BreathPlay Approach to Whole Life Fitness*, Ian Jackson coined the term "UpsideDown breathing" to describe the BreatheOutDynamic system with its active, spine-stretching outbreath and passive, relaxed inbreath—just the opposite of plain old breathing. BODs *is* the active, spine-stretching outbreath and the relaxed, passive inbreath. Trust nature's vacuum/suction and the elastic recoil of your chest and abdominal muscles to do the rest. Your whole body will be the beneficiary.

This is a revolutionary idea based on sound physics principles. (Read Chapter 2, "Building the Case for the BreatheOutDynamic system—Proof Is in Your BODy" for more information.) When you push air out, then relax, the same amount of air enters your body automatically and fast, without effort. Whether you have difficulty breathing or are a marathon runner, you have a net energy gain because you relaxed instead of sucking in air.

BODs SHAKES UP
THE VINAIGRETTE IN YOUR LUNGS

It may sound appropriate to be a chest breather — after all, your lungs are located in your chest. But, Josiah Child, MD, Chairman of Emergency Medicine at Los Alamos Medical Center in New Mexico, and a BODs athlete, clarifies this misnomer. "Chest breathing is ineffective," he says, "because it reduces the opportunity for oxygen to enter blood via capillaries, which surround the lungs like lace."

Dr. Child uses the metaphor of a cruet of oil and vinegar salad dressing. Unstirred, the lighter oil remains at the top, while the heavier vinegar is at the bottom. "It's definitely not ready to be served," he says. Now, in your mind, replace oil and vinegar with air and blood in the lungs. If you're a chest breather, lighter air is at the top; heavier blood is at the bottom, making it difficult for oxygen to transfer into the blood.

Child goes on to say, "Nuclear studies using 'tagged' (radioactive) gas and blood clearly show that blood often concentrates at the bottom of the lungs while air remains at the top. This goes unnoticed in our sedentary twenty-first century," he says, "unless you are sick or are exercising. It needs to be corrected because breathing is not just a matter of moving air and blood in and out but getting the two to mix effectively."

How do you get this mixing to happen? In the cruet it's easy. You shake it. In the human body, Child recommends using the BreatheOutDynamic system. "If you contract abdominal muscles as the first part of the outbreath, while creating some resistance to air leaving the lungs by using pursed lips, you force blood into the upper lobes prior to air leaving.

"By continuing to make the area around the lower lobes of the lungs smaller with your outbreath, you not only force air out of the lungs, but blood as well. This is what really creates the BODs vacuum. Blood is pushed out so that air rushes back into the lower lobes. The inbreath needs to be quick and coordinated because if you wait too long, blood will fill the lower lungs, competing with air for space. Once air is equally distributed in the lungs, blood, which is under higher pressure than air, is forced to distribute itself equally around the lungs.

"Now," says Child, "that's a nicely whisked lung vinaigrette, ready to go!"

If you want to improve the quality of your life, breathe slower—that is, use the BreatheOutDynamic system. Your heart and your lungs won't have to work so hard. Asian cultures teach that you have a certain number of breaths in your lifetime. You just don't know the number. In other words, efficiency counts.

I remember when I was first learning the BreatheOutDynamic system in 1987, following a weeklong workshop Ian Jackson taught at Omega Institute in Rhinebeck, New York. After two to three weeks of using BODs while walking, I was loving being *in* the outbreath because I discovered how quickly, easily, and passively air was entering my lungs. My body was saying thanks for getting rid of carbon dioxide and letting in oxygen without effort. As a result, I had more energy for walking. I was hooked on the BreatheOutDynamic system.

Understanding the connection between structure and function, and the difference between plain old breathing and the BreatheOutDynamic system, puts you on the road to developing a user-friendly body. Exercise will no longer be boring because you will be listening to your body. Interior discourse will replace exterior distractions like TV, cell phone, and iPod. Exercise will be easier because you can choreograph your daily routines using BODs principles. There is nothing to memorize, but you must practice. This is all based on your new understanding at the gut level, the level of your muscles.

Listen, observe, and practice to create awareness and respect for your amazing body.

INTEGRATION
EVERYTHING INFLUENCES EVERYTHING
RESPIRATORY SYSTEM MEETS AUTONOMIC NERVOUS SYSTEM

Breathing is wired into the human brain, as it was eons ago, even when brains were smaller. The breathing center is still located at the back of the neck in the brain stem below the skull, unprotected. This is the location of the connection between the breathing center and nerves of the autonomic nervous system (ANS). The ANS controls involuntary activities like heartbeat, intestinal contractions, and sweating. Your ANS also acts as a protective mechanism to help you deal with danger and then recover from that danger and get back to business as usual.

Today, the ANS still performs these duties. What has changed, and continues to change, is our environment. Today, perceived dangers are totally different than eons ago because our environment is totally different. The problem is that the ANS is still performing as if the car that cut you off on the turnpike was the feline jaguar lunging for your jugular. So you get revved up needlessly.

The task of the ANS, connected to the brain but separate from it, is to keep the human beast on an even keel, physiologically, emotionally, and functionally.

The ANS accomplishes this task using three nervous systems: the sympathetic, parasympathetic, and enteric. The sympathetic and parasympathetic nervous systems balance each other in their effects on the heart, lungs, viscera, and circulation—essential body systems required for survival. The sympathetic nervous system revs you up; the parasympathetic calms you down. Together they strive to create balance. The enteric nervous system exists in the gut and is largely independent of the ANS and central control by the brain. Thus, the belly has a "mind" of its own and is responsible for "gut" reactions, also known as intuition.

In today's stressful world, creating physiological balance is a complex yet simple pursuit, one that has been largely ignored. We aren't even aware that our bodies are stressed and on the brink of breakdown. We simply believe and act as if bodies can do all that we ask of them, without consequence.

"Western medicine and culture are dominated by the sympathetic nervous system that revs us up," says Dr. Will Evans, a family practice physician in Carbondale, Colorado, whose main interest is the heart. With the help of the owner of a Dallas, Texas, fitness club, BODs guru Ian Jackson met Dr. Evans in 2000. (Jackson told me this in a 2008 phone conversation.) During that encounter, Dr. Evans connected Jackson to a laptop computer via chest electrodes while he was running on a treadmill and, of course, focusing on the BreatheOutDynamic system. What Dr. Evans discovered shocked him. During this fast-paced exercise, Jackson was functioning with his parasympathetic nervous system — the part that promotes relaxation. Rather than being stressed, Jackson's heart and vital organs were basically at rest.

Based on this chance encounter, Dr. Evans told me in a phone interview in 2010, he is convinced that the BreatheOutDynamic system stimulates the parasympathetic nervous system.

The truth is that bodies *can* manage driving on the highway at 65 miles per hour, or faster, while the brain is talking on the telephone (illegal in some states) and scanning the radio dial to get the traffic report, even in rush-hour traffic in New Jersey. And indeed, the bodymind, a single, integrated unit, has extraordinary capabilities. The bodymind *can* work overtime and put up with a job you hate so you can pay the bills. But the cost is very high. Your energy and attention are drawn away from body messages, as well as meaningful personal relationships and responsibilities that can keep you on an even keel.

THE PERTINENCE
OF THE WORD *BODYMIND*

Candace Pert, PhD (1946–2014), biophysicist, psychopharmacologist, and author who understood and used the relaxation effect of the outbreath, wrote extensively about the bodymind as a unified whole. Everything is connected to everything, and thus everything influences everything. Just because your head sits on top of your body does not mean that it is more influential or more intelligent than what lies below. Yet in our culture, we live in our heads. We allow the brain to rule the body. We ignore body messages. The BreatheOutDynamic system helps you turn this upside down.

Pert's research reveals the connection between the chemicals of emotion, the mind, *and* the body. She acknowledges the innate intelligence of the body—its organs, muscles, fascia (connective tissue), and other tissues. The title of her audio book says it all: *Your Body Is Your Subconscious Mind* (Boulder, Colorado: Sounds True, 2000).

Pert admitted people's willingness to pop

pills for a quick fix, and that medications cause many health problems. In her book, *Molecules of Emotion: The Science Behind Mind-Body Medicine* (New York, New York: Simon & Schuster, 1998), she recommends taking action in three areas: first, what you eat; second, how you move; and third, what you think.

Pert includes breathing in the movement category. She notes that most people breathe too rapidly and shallowly, activating the sympathetic nervous system. This puts all parts of the human body under great stress. She says that breathing is not just about filling the lungs. Effective breathing, she explains, stimulates the spine and thus the entire nervous system, which includes neurotransmitters and hormones.

Just don't be surprised when your bodymind talks back to you with interrupted sleep; ineffective digestion, elimination, and reproduction; no energy; or a chronic or terminal disease. Gabor Maté, MD, validates this fact in vivid detail in his book, *When the Body Says No: Exploring the Stress-Disease Connection* (Hoboken, New Jersey: John Wiley & Sons, Inc., 2003).

Bodies do have their limits—but keep working until death do us part. When dysfunction occurs, people want a quick fix, and doctors want to satisfy their patients. The root cause—often an out-of-control ANS—is rarely considered.

To understand how the autonomic nervous system works, I think of a seesaw. One end—the sympathetic nervous system—revs you up, ready for an emergency. The other end of the seesaw—the parasympathetic nervous system—slows and calms you down.

I remember when I was a kid playing on a seesaw. My fear was always that I might be stuck up in the air, with the other kid's feet planted firmly on the ground. To prevent this I would moderate my own effort to keep a pleasing, gleeful balance of up-and-down movement (parasympathetic nervous system). I was afraid the other kid would create a wild and crazy scenario of fear and anxiety (sympathetic nervous system)—stuff that was familiar in my own family life. Sometimes it was a self-fulfilling prophecy—I did get stuck in the up position.

If only I had known the BreatheOutDynamic system when I was a kid. I really could have enjoyed being up high on that seesaw, knowing that my focused outbreath would help me stay relaxed. I wouldn't have given the other kid power over my existence. As a kid, of course, I would not have known anything about the parasympathetic nervous system. All I would have needed to know is that blowing out slowly would help me to relax, feel confident, and have fun.

And truly, that is all *you* need to know about how the ANS manages energy. As my respiratory home care patient Alma Alvarez observed, "I don't think you need to be a scientist to understand that breathing affects the nervous system. I learned this through experience. If you are breathing fast and shallow, you will feel anxious and exhausted. If this gets you bent out of shape, do the opposite to relax — focus on BODs." Unfortunately, it is not common knowledge that the active outbreath promotes relaxation.

For years, Ian Jackson said, and I have also, "The active outbreath promotes relaxation of the autonomic nervous system." But, I have yet to find this specifically spelled out in respiratory textbooks and mainstream health books. Why? There are many reasons. **FIRST:** Breathing is considered, even in the medical community, an unconscious process, one that keeps going until the day you die, without need for substantial definition or any personal awareness or intervention. **SECOND:** The general term "breathing" connotes inbreath, not outbreath. **THIRD:** Western culture and science consider the effect of breathing on the human body only when there is an emergency — and then drugs are given to control the breathing process. **FOURTH:** Most doctors are no longer teachers with practical solutions. **FIFTH:** Who would finance evidence-based scientific research to study the outbreath? Drug companies? The federal government?

OUT-OF-THE-BOX THINKING

Consider this not-so-off-the-wall notion that occurred to me as I was writing this book: Your eyes and ears are actually part of your respiratory system. What they see and hear can change your breathing.

Here's my out-of-the-box line of thinking: The eyes and ears, like the nose, mouth, and skin, are sensory organs. They transmit information about the outside environment to the environment inside your body. It is the job of the ANS (composed of parasympathetic and sympathetic nervous systems) to analyze this information in order to maintain homeostasis — the healthy, balanced state that keeps you on an even keel — or to prepare you for action. If you *see* something that is disturbing, like a flickering red glow in the next room, *hear* a crackling sound, then *smell* something acrid, your respiratory rate speeds up and your palms become sweaty.

By the time your body starts breathing fast, the nerves that connect your sensory organs to your brain have already done their job transferring information to your brain stem — the breathing center. Other nerves have processed the signals and alerted your muscles for action. The ANS, using all this sensory input, works quicker than you can imagine.

Then, you remember that you put dinner on the stove in the next room a long while ago.

When your body is revved up by the sympathetic nervous system—caused by shallow chest breathing or focusing only on the inbreath or seeing something disturbing—the resulting cascade of impulses and chemicals prepares your body, ironically, for survival, not action. Your body shunts blood to organs essential for survival—heart, lungs, and reproductive organs. The brain, the digestive system, and muscles do not receive blood.

So, your ability to think your way out of a situation may be limited. You may be exhausted and feel nauseous if you've just eaten. Some of these sympathetic nervous system chemicals are neurotransmitters, such as norepinephrine and acetylcholine, which act only within the nervous system. Others are released into the bloodstream, by definition becoming hormones, which can have a long-lasting impact on the entire body. Thus, living in your sympathetic nervous system can have detrimental effects, such as ineffective digestion, elimination, and reproduction, as well as fatigue, fuzzy thinking, and numbness.

People who use the BreatheOutDynamic system experience the effects of out-of-the-box thinking when their active, spine-stretching outbreath stimulates parasympathetic relaxation. Without BODs, stressful situations stimulate the energy-draining effects of the sympathetic nervous system. BODs calming effect on the nervous system has not been studied extensively. Rather, this knowledge is the result of astute observation, which, after all, is the first step in any scientific exploration.

Reality Check
Expanding Your BODs practice

1. What is it about BODs that piques your interest?
2. What muscles become strong when you practice BODs?
3. How do you use BODs for energy and relaxation?

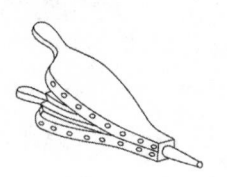

FITTING BODS INTO YOUR LIFE

CHAPTER 5

THE NEXT STEP

USING *BODs* WITH MOVEMENT

"We should go to school for breathing and walking."
Philippe Petit,
high-wire artist

"Rhythm is born in all of us."
Ginger Rogers,
actress and director

Now that you have learned and practiced the two-step basics of the BreatheOutDynamic system and understand its simplicity, you are ready to learn how to design your own BODs experience to suit your body's varying needs as you move. Your design is based on the basic BODs principle: *the outbreath empowers you.*

THE BREATHEOUTDYNAMIC SYSTEM AS MUSIC

Human beings are innately musical. In the womb we experience our mother's breathing and feel her heart beating. It is constant. It is a hug and the beat of a drum. And then, suddenly, we are on our own. We have our own built-in hug and rhythm. Both are incessant. They require no thought and often go unnoticed—for years. They influence us—always. The BreatheOutDynamic system asks you to be aware of your body's music.

BODs rhythms help you organize your physical activities to foster body, mind, and spirit harmony. By counting steps used for each outbreath and each inbreath (one breathing cycle), you actually measure the amount of energy you need for specific tasks.

Here's how you start to discover your rhythms when exercising, whether sitting in a chair alternately lifting your feet or slowly walking outside or on a treadmill. Count *in your head* the number of steps you take while blowing out and then the number of steps you take while letting in air. The numbers do not have to be consistent from breathing cycle to breathing cycle. It is *not* the numbers by themselves that matter. What is important is the effect they have on your body. Your goal is to support your activity with adequate energy— air. Remember, you gain strength from your outbreath. Generally, your outbreath wants to be about twice as long as your inbreath. However, you can play around with the length of your outbreath. Let your inbreath be as short as possible, so that you can return to the strength-giving outbreath. With practice, you may be comfortable with an outbreath that's three or more times as long as your inbreath. Let your body be your guide. With time, you'll be amazed at how good a really long outbreath feels.

Counting is meditation—deep focus on the moment that you are experiencing right now. Thus, the BreatheOutDynamic system turns walking or any exercise into moving meditation with all the benefits, and maybe more, of stationary meditation.

When I walk in my neighborhood, my BODs rhythm is often 7 steps during the outbreath and 2 steps (7-2) during the inbreath. Sometimes it is 5-2 or even 10-3. I like to play around with the numbers to see how different rhythms make me feel. When hiking up a mountain, I'm always changing my rhythm and pace, depending on the ups and downs. Going up, my rhythm might be 3-2 or even 2-1, helping air to come into my body more often to energize my vigorous activity. Going down requires less energy, so I can increase the length of my outbreath. I still count in my head and focus on the BreatheOutDynamic system because it relaxes my bodymind and allows me to be a kid again, hopping from rock to rock, being light-footed in the forest.

With BODs, I am the musician mountain climber. I create the rhythm. I create the harmony. I get to the top of the mountain with joy—no shortness of breath, no cramps, no heavy legs. My body is at peace, ready for the next mountain.

Creating your own rhythm is the playful art of the BreatheOutDynamic system. You have all the answers right there within your own body. Experiment with different rhythms, different tempos. Let your mind listen to your body. Honor its messages. Challenge your body. Take it to the edge. Look around. Discover what the word *comfortable* means to you. Your body will tell you. Tomorrow your body may tell you something different. The BreatheOutDynamic system helps you grow, adapt to change, and meet your goals.

LESSONS FROM ATHLETES

Ian Jackson was an eclectic athlete — surfer, dancer, runner, cyclist, swimmer, and adventurer. He ran marathons, competed in the Ironman triathlon three times, and coached Olympic and Tour de France cycling teams.

While developing the BreatheOutDynamic system more than forty years ago, Jackson discovered that elite, competitive cyclists who were prone to leg injuries would hurt the same leg repeatedly. When he contemplated the rhythm of breathing and pedal-stroke movement, he thought about the 4/4 marching cadence, which is four beats to a measure — hup, two, three, four. The first beat is strongest. The second is weak; the third is strong but not as strong as the first; and the fourth beat is weak. Knowing this, Jackson realized that this ingrained 4/4 marching rhythm was creating cycling injuries because the same leg would experience the strong demands of strong pedal strokes. Using a tape measure, he measured the calf muscles of injured cyclists. The injured leg generally had a calf muscle that was larger than the other because it was the leg working on the strong first and third beats.

Using these observations about calf-muscle size, Jackson designed a unique breathing rhythm that he intuitively understood would solve the problem. He called this rhythm SwitchSide breathing. It depends upon outbreath and inbreath steps or pedal strokes adding up to an odd number, as opposed to the standard 4/4 time, which adds up to an even number.

SwitchSide breathing allows the first step or stroke of each breathing cycle to change from one leg to the other. Thus natural stresses of movement are equalized between both legs. When Jackson followed up with the injured athletes, who had been using BODs SwitchSide breathing for a few months, he observed that individual athletes' calf muscles were equal in size, and injuries were not as frequent.

SwitchSide Breathing
Rhythms, Numbers, and Movement

Whether or not you are able to exercise at a fast pace, start coordinating the BreatheOutDynamic system with movement while walking slowly. This gives your muscles time to learn BODs and your brain time to develop respect for the intelligence of your muscles.

Let's take a walk counting steps. First, figure out your own walking rhythm. You want to know how many steps you take during the outbreath and how many during the inbreath. You can either assign some numbers, such as 3 steps for the outbreath and 2 for the inbreath (3–2), or just start using BODs, counting in your head to determine the number of steps you actually take for the outbreath and inbreath.

Whichever method you choose, you need to play around with the numbers. Find the numbers that make your movement effortless. You can use a different set of numbers for every breathing cycle or use the same numbers. When you add the outbreath number and the inbreath number together, the sum should be an odd number. This numerical trick of SwitchSide breathing saves wear and tear on muscles and joints. Counting steps is the way to measure the amount of air you need, depending upon what you're doing—the way of letting your brain listen to your body and honor its messages. This is truly moving meditation.

REALITY CHECK
EXPANDING YOUR BODs PRACTICE

1. What are your BODs SwitchSide breathing rhythms?
2. What adventures will BODs help you achieve?
3. How is SwitchSide breathing changing your activities?

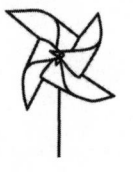

CHAPTER 6

BECOMING YOUR OWN PERSONAL TRAINER

"When you arise in the morning, think of what a
privilege it is to be alive — to breathe,
to think, to enjoy, to love."
Marcus Aurelius,
Roman emperor

"Exercise is so boring. I can only do it when I watch TV."

"Walking is only fun when I'm listening to my iPod."

Are these your words?

Are you looking for exercise that's more stimulating and effective?

Would you like to tap into your own inner music?

It makes no difference whether or not you use modern technology, go to the gym, or exercise outside. In this chapter, you'll find energizing new ideas to move yourself toward your fitness goals.

THE BreatheOutDynamic system AND Personal Power

The BreatheOutDynamic system puts *you* in charge of your body. You can choreograph your movements with your breath as you go along. There's no need to remember which part of the exercise requires outbreath or inbreath. Simply follow the basic BODs principle: The outbreath empowers you. Therefore *exhale on exertion.* However, this does require listening carefully to your body. Forget the TV or iPod. Don't even think of multitasking. Exercise combined with BODs requires your undivided attention.

Why should you exhale on exertion? Remember the bellows that pushes air out to fan the fire? Your fire is your metabolism, the internal body combustion that energizes you. It's the BODs outbreath that fans your metabolic fire. And all this time you and everybody else have been thinking that taking *in* air is what breathing is all about.

No, it's just the opposite.

You can prove this basic BODs principle, that the outbreath gives you power (the ability to do work), by testing your muscles, a process called kinesiology. Use the following resistance exercise to ask your muscles for information. Here's the question: Which gives you more strength—outbreath or inbreath? Muscles are smart and expressive. By doing this resistance experiment, you can observe and experience the answer.

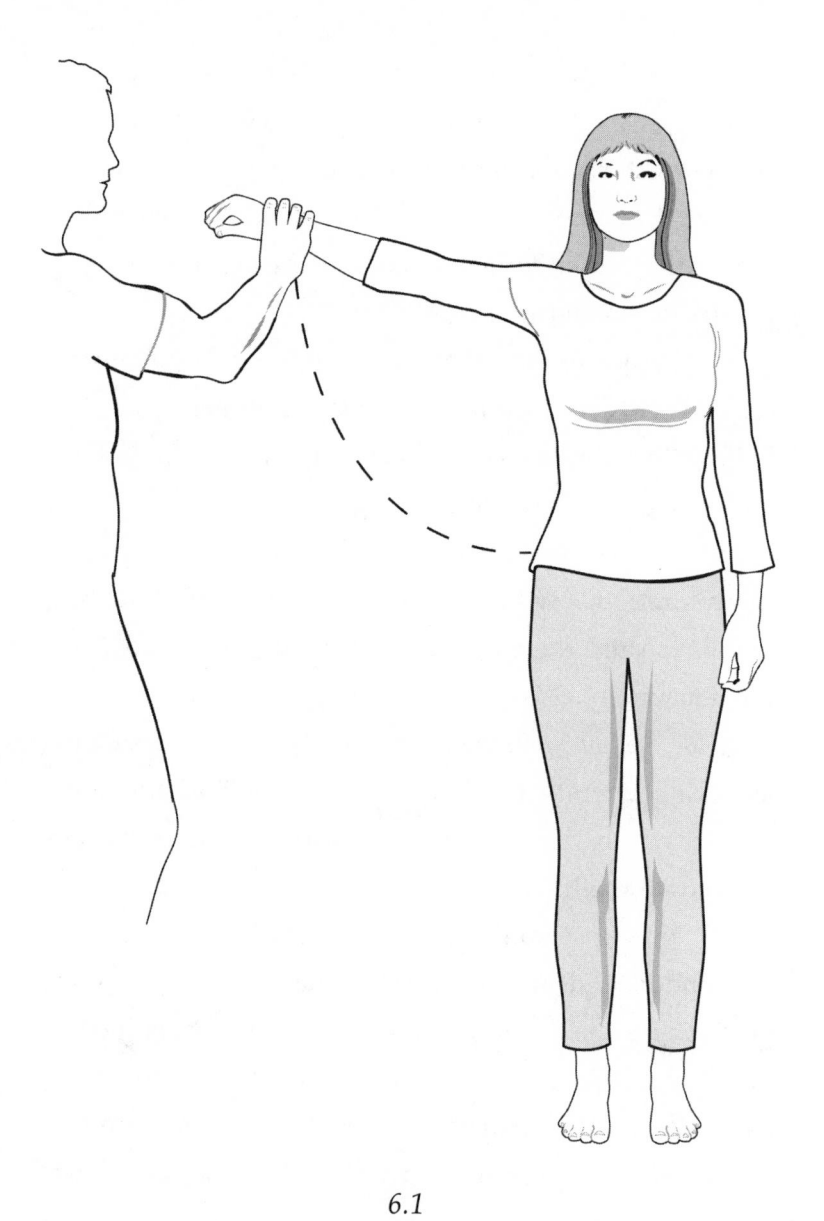

6.1

In this kinesiology experiment, the tester (left) and resister discover which part of the breathing cycle – outbreath or inbreath – generates strength. Follow instructions in the text.

Here's how the test works. It requires two players and is really a game of discovery, not competition. You be the resister, your partner the tester. The resister stands or sits tall with one arm stretched out sideways, slightly higher than shoulder level, palm facing down. The tester pushes down on the resister's wrist.

The job of the resister is to oppose this downward force. Try it, and see how it goes. Now, here's the test. Follow the above instructions twice more, first while taking *in* air; then while blowing *out*.

Observe what happens. When did you experience more strength — with inbreath or outbreath? You may have expected the inbreath to provide power to resist, but amazingly, it's just the opposite: *It's the outbreath that gives you more strength.* Most people define breathing as taking air into the body. BODs redefines breathing as the active, spine-stretching outbreath and passive, relaxed inbreath.

Now that you've done this resistance experiment, you understand in your muscles that efficient, effective breathing is the act of pushing out air and *letting* it come in again. The bonus is that the completed outbreath automatically creates a vacuum inviting the same amount of air back into your lungs. Thus, *BODs emphasizes a long, active outbreath.* The length of your outbreath is your decision, based on what you're doing and the messages your body is giving you.

In the beginning of this resistance experiment, did you do a breath-hold? If you kept your lips tight together or grimaced, you were holding your breath, keeping old air locked inside your body. This gives muscles a false sense of strength with a high cost: increased blood pressure and decreased blood flow, especially in and around lung tissue. With a BODs gentle, active, spine-stretching outbreath, you achieve strength safely.

I have used this demonstration for years and discovered that even people who consider themselves weak are amazed by the strength they have during the outbreath. People who are very strong are equally amazed that their strength can be overcome during their *inbreath* – when *everyone* is inherently weak.

Now translate this new awareness into action. For example, if you are short of breath climbing stairs, exhale while doing the hard work of climbing; then briefly pause with both feet on one step to let in air. Then resume blowing out while climbing, pausing for the inbreath. Listen to your body to decide how many stairs to climb during one outbreath. Your goal is to reach the top of the stairs without shortness of breath – a benefit of the BreatheOutDynamic system.

Exercise will never be boring or tedious again. Now you have your body to watch and listen to instead of TV or your iPod. With BODs, you are the most important part of the learning equation. You have the questions, and your body—your teacher—reveals the answers, if you listen.

Your Body as Teacher

Because the BreatheOutDynamic system lets you be the choreographer, you can exercise within *your* limits, deciding which exercises are appropriate for *you*. But just because you are able to do an exercise or stretch does not mean it's beneficial. Your body will reveal this information, either immediately or over time.

My body spoke to me after a trip to India in 2005. During my visit I learned a yoga routine. I was careful to do only the moves that my body could do—not all those that my instructor's body could do.

This yoga routine enlivened me. After I returned home, I continued to do yoga several times a week. Six months later, I was having difficulty getting out of my new car. My legs and hips were just not working right. At first I thought it must be the car seat because I was driving five hundred miles a week. I tried all sorts of different seat adjustments, but the problem persisted. Then climbing stairs became painful. I realized I had to think differently—to consider how *I* was contributing to the problem.

I examined my exercise routine and decided to change one thing. I stopped trying to touch my toes when seated on the floor with my legs stretched out in front of me. I imagined that I had been overstretching my low back and hip muscles. I heard their complaints as pain, the pain of being irritated and inflamed, much like arthritis. So I stopped that stretch. Slowly over the next few months, the condition corrected itself, exonerating my car seat.

This potentially crippling experience reminded me why I had quit running thirty years ago. For a few years I had been running 3 to 5 miles three or four times a week. Then I began experiencing hip pain upon rising from a seated position. Thinking that the problem was caused by the impact of road running, I quit. Walking coordinated with BODs became my daily exercise. About a year later, I was pain-free.

Now, I am revisiting this overuse injury of long ago. I remember stretching the back of my legs on the hip-high stone wall near my house. I was doing what I had seen other runners doing: stretching before, during, and after a run. In effect, I was irritating the same tissues as my recent yoga stretch.

Here's the moral of the story. There is always something new to learn about yourself, and it's never too late to *listen to your body*. Thanks be to BODs, with its emphasis on awareness, for teaching me this lesson — over and over again.

EXPANDING YOUR BODS SKILLS

Each day for a week or so, spend 15 to 20 minutes or more teaching your muscles the BreatheOutDynamic system. (Refer to basic BODs concepts in Chapter 3.) Muscles are smart but require practice in order to perform consistently. I recommend that you first learn BODs either sitting or lying down before using it with movement. Increase the frequency or duration when you feel ready. Don't be surprised if at first your belly muscles don't respond. You may need to press your hands gently on your belly for the outbreath and release them for the inbreath. Soon your belly muscles will get the idea.

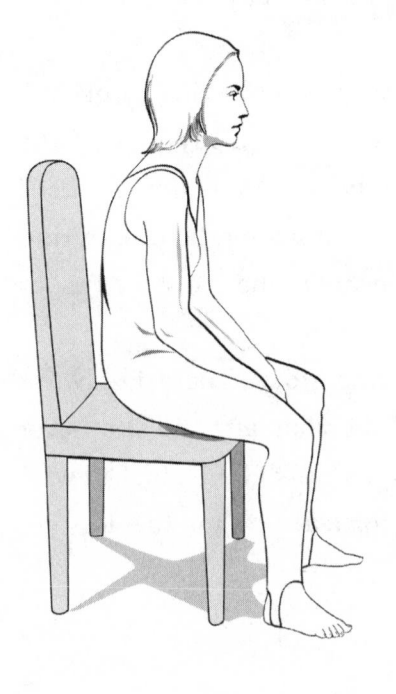

6.2a

With slouched posture, notice rounded shoulders, head in front of body, and caved-in chest, which prevents lung expansion.

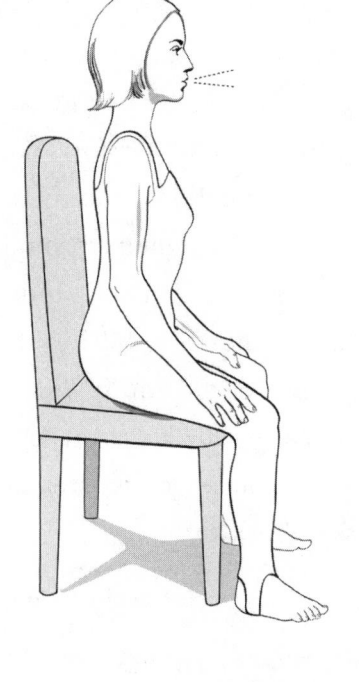

6.2b

With ideal posture, notice ears over shoulders, chest out, and shoulders over hips with feet flat on the floor. Also notice the normal curve behind the neck (cervical spine) and in the low back (lumbar spine). When standing, head and shoulders should be over feet.

Good posture is important, whether you choose to stand, sit, or lie down to learn BODs. Ideal posture is to stand or sit tall and stick out your chest, with your ears over your shoulders. If you are standing, your shoulders should be in line with your hips and feet. Pretend that marionette-puppet strings extend from the top of your head, pulling you up tall. If you are sitting, rest your relaxed hands on your thighs and place your feet flat on the floor—no crossed legs. If you are lying in bed or on the floor, on your back or side, you may want to bend your knees for comfort. Position yourself as close to these ideal postures as possible, without pain or strain.

Now you are ready to focus on basic BODs.

Simply blow out gently using your lips, tongue, or teeth to restrict the outflow of air while contracting your belly, like closing a bellows. You're not trying to blow out all the air in your lungs. Blow out to a point of comfort. You decide what's enough. For the inbreath, *let* the air in through your nose, or if your nose is clogged, through your mouth. (See Chapter 4 sidebar "The Perils of Mouth Breathing.") There is absolutely no need to help in the air. Learn to trust that the amount of air you blew out is sucked back in when you release your belly muscles. This is a response to the vacuum you have just created. It's the way our universe works. Trust it.

ALTERNATE NOSTRIL BREATHING

While BODs major focus is on the active outbreath through gently pursed lips, it is essential to keep nasal passages open so air can flow freely. Everyone needs to clean out their nasal passages regularly—some people more than others.

When the sinuses, small air-filled cavities inside your head around your nose and eyes, become clogged with mucus, you feel nagging facial pressure. To eliminate this, try alternate nostril breathing, a yoga technique that utilizes the forceful, flowing outbreath and the passive, instantaneous inbreath.

Here's how to do the technique. Using thumb and index finger, block your nostrils alternately. Press your thumb against one nostril to close it, then exhale through the open nostril. With your index finger, close the nostril from which you just exhaled. Release your thumb. In that instant of release, air is sucked into your body. Now exhale through that newly opened nostril. For a minute or two, continue this rhythmic activity of blocking and blowing, using BODs. Observe that air comes in—fast. That's how nature's vacuum works.

Blow your nose as needed. Notice all the junk that you expel. Do this alternate-nostril-breathing routine once or twice a day, or as often as necessary to relieve sinus pressure. Soon—probably within a week or a month or two—you will be able to breathe effectively through your nose.

When using BODs quietly in a stationary position, it's preferable to let air in through your nose to allow it to act as filter, humidifier, and temperature regulator. However, during activity it can be hard to get adequate air in through your nose, so it's helpful, not harmful, to leave your mouth open a bit when using BODs.

Remember, *effort is needed for the outbreath. No effort is needed for the inbreath.* In that instant when you release your belly muscles, fresh air rushes in.

Feel the rhythm that you establish with each cycle of outbreath and inbreath. Be right there with your lungs and your belly, experiencing their responses.

BODs Spinal Stretch

Stretching your entire spine is essential for its full function, which includes transmitting information to and from all parts of your body, via nerve fibers, chemical transmitters, and cerebrospinal fluid. The *lumbar stretch* is part of every basic BODs active outbreath. For feedback about where your lumbar spine is during each breathing cycle, use the back of a straight-backed chair or the flat surface of a wall, bed, or floor. When you contract your belly muscles for the outbreath, your lumbar spine moves closer to the back of the chair or flat surface of the wall, bed, or floor. When you release your belly muscles to let in air, the normal curve returns to your lumbar spine — it moves *away* from the chair back or flat surface. Your spine craves this movement of ebb — outbreath — and flow — inbreath. This is half of the BODs Spinal Stretch and is inherent in every BODs cycle.

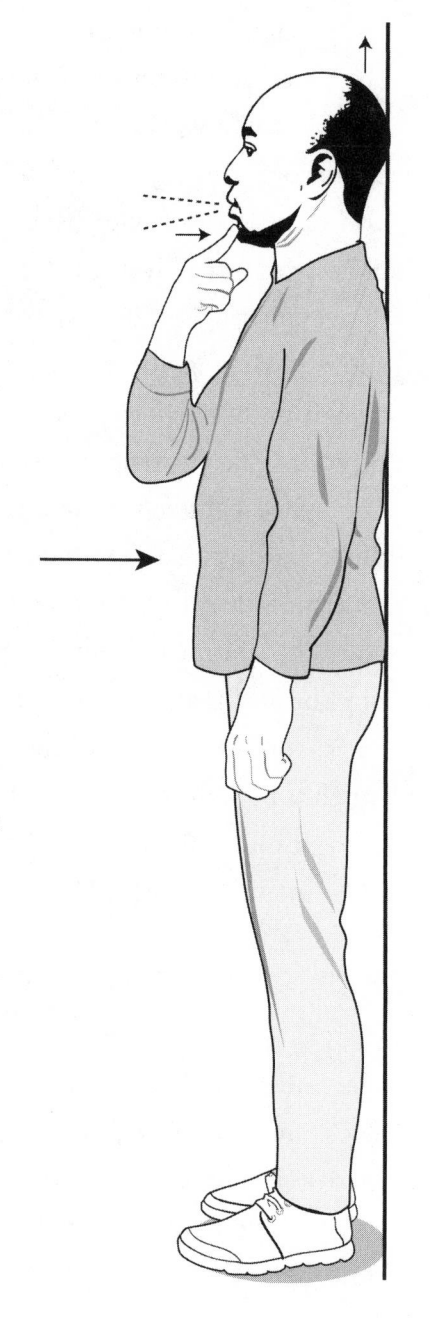

6.3

*To create the Chin-Tuck Full
Spinal Stretch, move the chin
down toward the collarbone
during the active outbreath.
Notice the crown of the head
moving up when the belly
is crunched. These actions
decrease the curve of both
cervical and lumbar parts of
the spine, creating the Full
Spinal Stretch.*

Here's the other half of the BODs Spinal Stretch. To stretch your *cervical spine*, do a Chin Tuck, achieved by gently moving your chin down toward the "V" in your collarbone during your active outbreath. This is not a nod or bowing of your head. Rather, your head remains over your shoulders as described in the ideal posture image (6.2b). For feedback about where your cervical spine is during the Chin Tuck, do it standing against a wall or lying in bed. You will experience the crown of your head moving up as you move your chin down. The space between your neck and the flat surface will decrease during the stretch (outbreath), with the curve returning during the passive inbreath when you release your chin. Hold this gentle stretch only for the duration of your outbreath. Repeat a few times.

Bodies in the twenty-first century spend far too much time locked in chairs. Use BODs Spinal Stretch for a few minutes throughout the day to provide stimulating movement that a healthy spine requires.

BODs Full Body Stretch

The Full Body Stretch, done lying down, combines Chin Tuck and Toe Tweak during the active outbreath. Toe Tweak is the gentle flexing (bending) of your ankles, bringing your toes toward your upper body during the outbreath. Feel your heels move in the opposite direction.

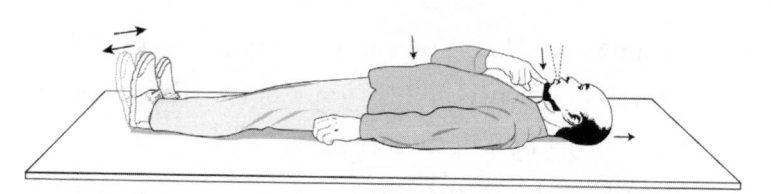

6.4

To create the Chin-Tuck Toe-Tweak Full Body Stretch while lying down, turn the Spinal Stretch into the Full Body Stretch by adding the Toe Tweak. Pull toes gently toward the knees during the long, slow outbreath as the chin moves gently toward the collarbone. For the inbreath, relax foot, belly, and neck muscles.

When simultaneously doing Chin Tuck and Toe Tweak, you are gently stretching your entire spine and the back of your legs.

Do this for a few minutes before getting out of bed. Consider staying in bed and doing the following exercises choreographed with BODs.

YOUR DAILY EXERCISE ROUTINE WITH BODs

Exercise, like sleep, should happen every day. Would you ever consider sleeping only three or four nights a week? Would you believe anyone who said sleeping is required only three or four nights a week? Of course not. Using BODs helps you look forward to exercising every day.

Exercising first thing in the morning is a beautiful

way to start your day. You can begin right in bed. BODs gently awakens every cell in your body. This is a fine time to do some Full Body Stretches.

With a bit more effort, you can move your entire body with the routine called Roll Over. You start exercising on your back, then continue by rolling over onto one side, then to your belly, then to the other side. If your bed is soft and bouncy, consider exercising on the floor. For comfort, you can use small pillows under your head and knees. Each of the following parts of Roll Over is done with the rhythmic accompaniment of BODs.

ROLL OVER ON YOUR BACK
Leg lifts and upside-down bicycles
strengthen your legs and
everything connected.

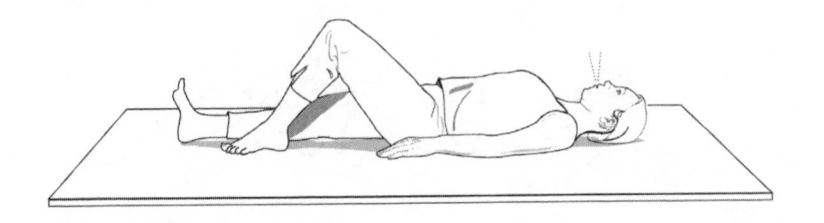

6.5a

Leg-lifts ready position illustrates how to safely start Roll Over when lying flat on your back. From this flat, bent-knee ready position, the straight leg is lifted slowly and to a comfortable height, then brought down slowly. Exercising legs one at a time protects the low back and provides rest time.

So there you are, lying on your back, exiting from sleep. You have been using BODs for a few minutes already. Now it's time to throw off the covers and move your limbs and joints.

LEG LIFTS are done s l o w l y *one leg at a time*, with the stationary leg bent with foot flat on the bed or floor. You'll notice that this avoids back strain. Lifting within your ability is what's important, not the height of your leg lift. Thus, a lift of several inches is beneficial. Your goal is to lift higher and higher when you are able. Lifting up is work. So exhale as you lift, then quickly let in the air. Exhale again while slowly lowering your leg. This, too, is work. You are resisting gravity to prevent your leg from slamming on the bed or floor. The outbreath supports this slow downward movement, and your tight belly muscles protect your low back. If or when you are able, you can move your leg up and down using one outbreath, establishing a new rhythm. Do these lifts until you notice fatigue or a heavy feeling, not to be confused with pain. Then do one or two more lifts. Working a little beyond your limit builds muscle tissue. You don't need to count repetitions, just stay focused on BODs, alert for your body's fatigue message. Your intention is to be with your muscles and feel them work. Know that your outbreath is powering them.

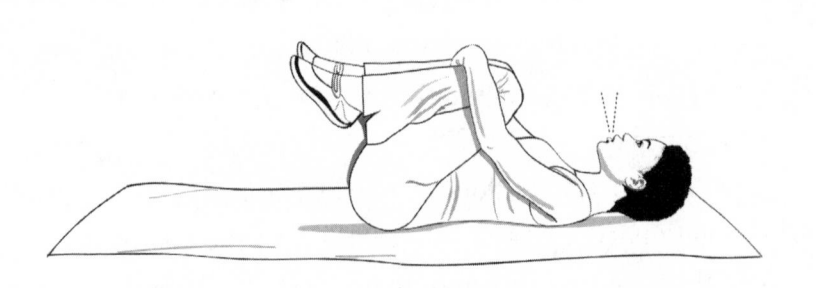

6.5b

Upside-down-bicycles ready position demonstrates how to start another part of Roll Over on your back. This leg-hug ready position is essential to prevent back strain. **If you are not able to maintain this position, wait to do bicycles until you can hug your legs.**

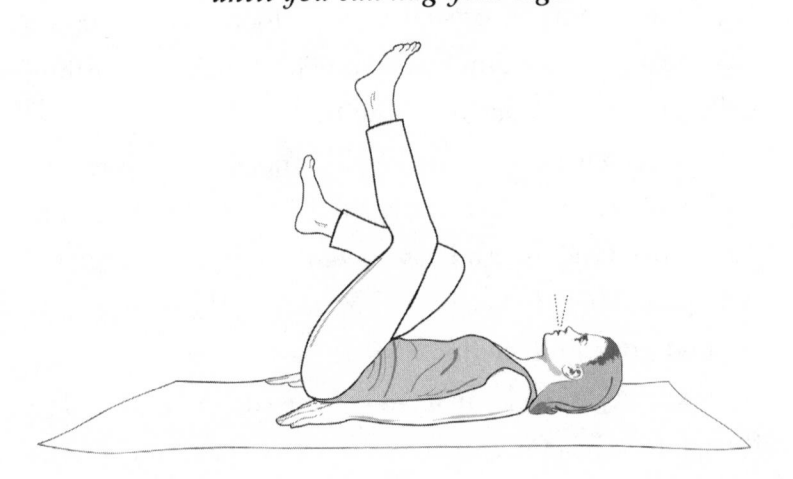

6.5c

While riding the upside-down bicycle, pedal forward or backward – go anywhere.

UPSIDE-DOWN BICYCLES are another exercise done while on your back, knees bent, feet in the air over your hips. To get in this position safely while on your back, start by wrapping your arms around your bent knees. *If you're not able to do this, wait to do these upside-down bicycles until you've become more flexible.* This bent-leg hug ensures that the weight of your legs is supported by your torso, not suspended over thin air, which will cause back pain.

Now pretend you are pedaling an upside-down bike. Feel the movement of your low back as you exhale on exertion. Your spine flattens, coming closer to the bed or floor. As you release your belly muscles for the inbreath, feel the curve in your spine return as your low back moves up, away from the flat surface. This is BODs powerful lumbar stretch, essential for back health.

When your legs start getting heavy, do a few more cycles, then stop. This sensation of heaviness is your body's message that enough is enough—it applies to all muscles. If you wish, you can do a different Roll Over exercise, then return to bicycles. By increasing the repetitions of slow exercise, you build endurance, which is actually more important than building strength with hard, fast exercise.

Maintaining a Healthy Back

In the process of getting older, people often complain about "my aching back." Guess what? BODs will help your aching back. The best strategy is to learn the BreatheOutDynamic system and use its active, spine-stretching outbreath with exercise and activities of daily living. While using BODs, you'll be building strong belly muscles—known in jock language as abs—which protect your low back. Forget sit-ups and curl-ups that can injure your back.

And forget back belts. The National Institute for Occupational Safety and Health studied their effectiveness with retail workers and found no evidence that wearing back belts reduced back injury or pain, as reported in the December 6, 2000, issue of the *Journal of the American Medical Association*. Here's the solution. When lifting anything, immediately start using the BreatheOutDynamic system—exhaling as you lift, or whistling while you work.

To determine your BODs rhythm while doing upside-down bicycles, count how many strokes (one stroke is one push of one foot) you can comfortably do during the outbreath. Allow 1 to 3 strokes for the inbreath. For example, your breathing cycle might look like this: Exhale for 4 strokes; let air in for 1 stroke. Your BODs rhythm is 4-1. Or, consider an outbreath of 6 strokes and an inbreath of 3 strokes, 6-3. You decide your BODs rhythm based on your activity, speed, and body messages.

The faster you pedal your imaginary bike and the harder you work, the more frequently you need to let in air. You accomplish this by changing the length of both outbreath and inbreath. Thus, the total length of each breathing cycle shortens, with the outbreath still remaining longer than the inbreath; for instance, 2-1. Change your breathing cycle numbers as often as you need, to avoid shortness of breath, boredom, or screeching to a halt.

To challenge different muscles, you can cycle in reverse as well as forward. The pace is your choice. Remember that slow exercise is very effective. For another challenge, especially for your brain, train one leg to cycle forward and the other to cycle backward—at the same time. Tip: Practice each leg separately before combining the opposing motions, like practicing a new piano piece one hand at a time.

ROLL OVER ON YOUR SIDE

Leg lifts and knee lifts improve your balance.

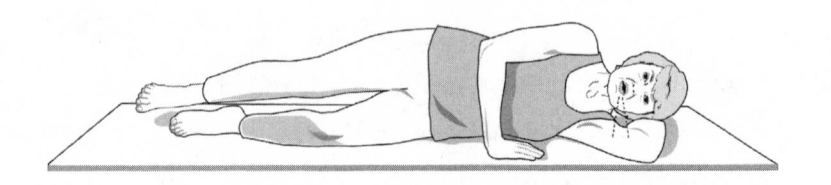

6.5d

This is ready position for Roll Over on either side. Head rests on bent arm. Legs are straight, one on top of the other, or with bottom leg slightly bent for stability.

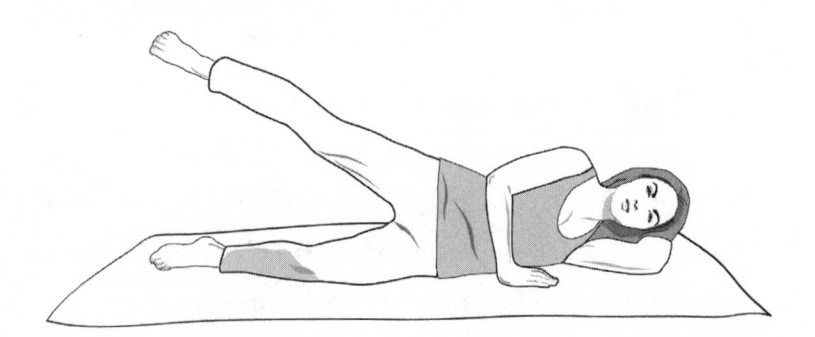

6.5e

For the scissor lift, raise top leg only as high as is comfortable. Daily practice of this exercise on both sides expands flexibility and balance.

Next, *roll over onto your side* to strengthen the muscles on the sides of your legs that influence your balance. Bend your bottom arm to cradle your head. Let your top arm gently fold over your belly so your hand can stabilize you, if needed. Your bottom leg is slightly bent. Slowly lift your top, straight leg, then lower it to the bed or floor. It's like opening and closing a scissor. How will you know when enough is enough? Your body will tell you.

Here's a variation that activates other muscles: Bend your top leg and hook your foot behind the knee of your slightly bent, bottom leg. Lift your top knee toward the sky, within your ability, then lower it to touch the flat surface, while focused on BODs. Do not roll your body as you lift your knee since this limits the effectiveness of the knee lift. Feel all the different muscles being gently activated, especially in your inner thigh. Again, the number and height of leg or knee lifts is your choice, based on your body messages. Figure out your basic BODs rhythm. As you progress, this knowledge helps you change pace and/or increase repetitions and the height of your leg or knee lifts.

Repeat these exercises on your other side after you complete the belly routine in the next section.

ROLL OVER ON YOUR BELLY
This strengthens legs,
low back, and everything connected.

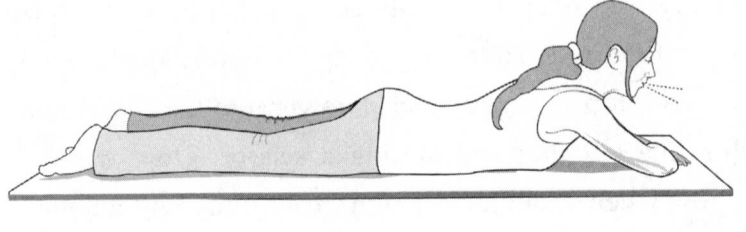

6.5f

This is ready position for Roll Over on belly. Shoulders are
raised comfortably with hands and forearms flat on the floor.

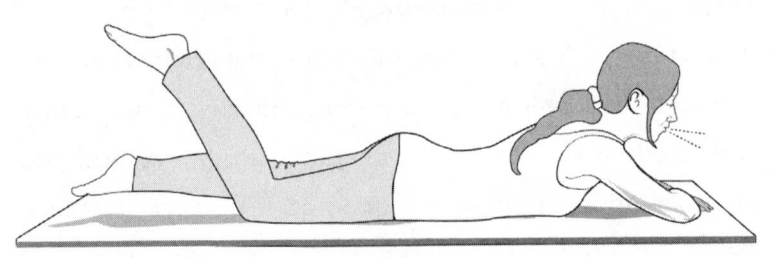

6.5g

When doing leg (calf) lifts on the belly, knees and thighs
remain on flat surface throughout the exercise.
Read text for instructions.

At this point, you're ready to roll onto your belly.
Lift your head, bend your arms, and support your torso
on your forearms, if you can. Otherwise lie flat and put

your head on the bed or floor, turning your head to the side or keeping it straight, with arms and hands in a comfortable position under your head or at your sides.

The action here is with your *lower legs*. Keep your thighs on the bed or floor. Bend your knees with your feet in the air, so that your lower legs are at right angles to your thighs. Lower your feet to the flat surface, then raise them again — like kicking when swimming. You can raise both legs together or one at a time. Or try hooking one foot on top of the opposite ankle and lifting. Now your top leg acts as a weight for the lower leg.

Although you are not moving your arms and your torso, they are working hard to support you. Experiment with your body position and BODs rhythm.

ROLL OVER ON YOUR OTHER SIDE
Repeat leg and knee lifts.

To wrap up your exercise session, turn to your other side and repeat Roll-Over-on-your-side exercises as previously described. When you're finished, roll to your back and simply focus on BODs for a minute or two as you assess your body from top to bottom and side to side. Imagine that with your outbreath you are directing oxygen to specific parts of your body, to thank your responsive muscles and joints. Be at peace with your body.

ROLLING OUT OF BED OR RISING OFF THE FLOOR

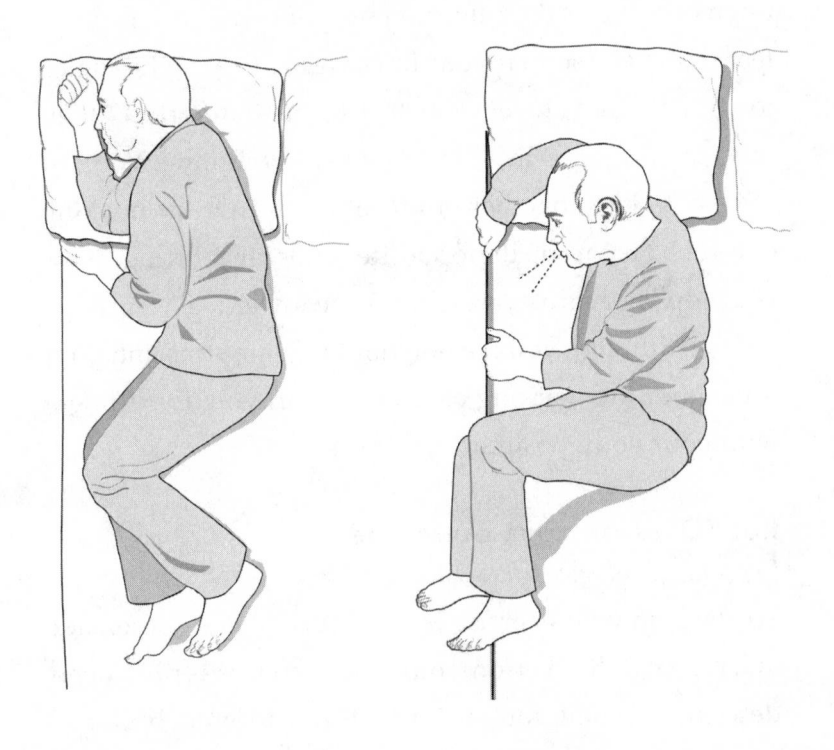

6.6a

Lying in bed, review how to use BODs to comfortably rise out of bed. Precise instructions are in the text.

6.6b

Exhale while rolling from lying down in bed to sitting upright at the edge of the bed.

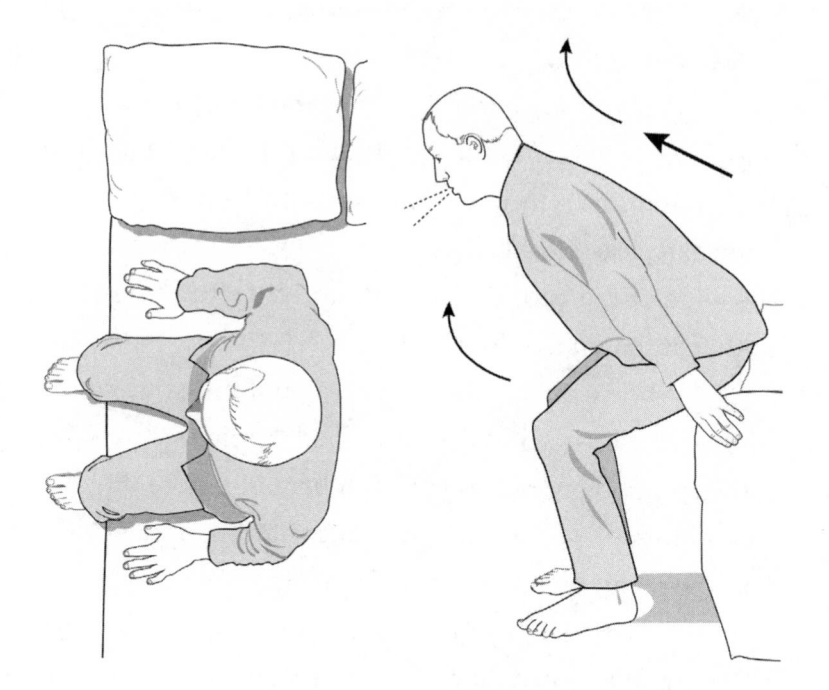

6.6c

*While sitting at
the edge of the bed,
visualize the next
action and breathing
cycle. Details are in
the text.*

6.6d

*Exhale to glide up to
standing position. Stand
tall, assess posture, and
make adjustments.*

When you are ready to roll out of bed or rise off the floor, here's how to do it efficiently while protecting your back. With every move you make, support your low back with the BODs active, spine-stretching outbreath and passive inbreath. Choreograph BODs with your every move to suit your need for energy. To review basic BODs, refer to Chapter 3.

If you're on your bed, exhale and roll to your side and face the edge. Let in air. While exhaling again, use hands and arms to push yourself up. Again, let in air. Then exhale as you bend your knees and swing them over the edge of the bed, rising to an upright sitting position with feet flat on the floor.

While exhaling, lean forward and use your hands to push against your thighs or bed, initiating upward movement. Then, rise to your full height. Before moving, focus on your posture for several breathing cycles. Now you are ready to move forward and start your day.

If you're on the floor, exhale, roll to your side, and let in air. While exhaling again, use your hands to push your torso up so you can shift into a kneeling position. During your next exhale, place one foot flat on the floor. With hands pushing down against your bent knee and the floor, exhale again and rise to a standing position. Choreograph your movements with BODs to suit your special needs, remembering to exhale on exertion.

CHAIR WALK
No-excuses fitness activity

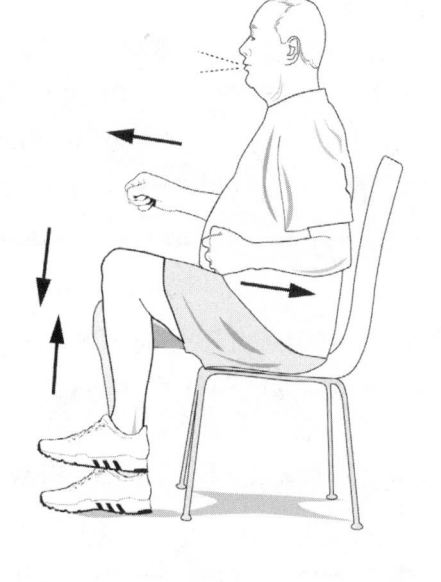

6.7

Chair Walk is done from the comfort and protection of a straight-backed chair. Explore movement possibilities with arms and legs.

If you live a sedentary lifestyle, have never exercised, or are debilitated from an accident, illness, or being overmedicated, you may *think* you cannot exercise because you believe that exercise will create shortness of breath, heavy legs, or cramps. This mindset actually promotes weakness. The BreatheOutDynamic system combined with chair exercise enlivens your body, promoting strength.

The human body needs to be moved every day—use it or lose it. In general, chair exercise is slow and deliberate, not fast paced. Exercise pushes waste products out of joints and muscles into the bloodstream for eventual removal. BODs should be an integral part of all exercise, helping you focus on your body, keeping you safe from overuse and injury. Find a straight-backed chair, and let's get started.

Wiggle your butt into the back of the chair and feel your spine against it. First, do a few BODs cycles. Notice how your spine moves toward the back of the chair with your outbreath and away from the chair with your inbreath. This is BODs lumbar stretch, explained previously in this chapter. Now you're ready to start your actual Chair Walk.

LEGS are not only important for movement through space but also for flow of blood back to the heart. Pretend that you are walking. Exhale and lift one foot to a comfortable height; then quickly let in air. Exhale as your foot slowly returns to the floor. Repeat with the other foot. Develop a deliberate, comfortable routine. To expand your abilities, you can raise and lower your foot with one outbreath. Or, see how many leg lifts you can do without shortness of breath or other signs of fatigue before you stop exhaling. Your body will tell you when it needs more energy — when it's time to let air in, and then to start another BODs cycle.

ARMS, involved in upper body strength and balance, need to be exercised also. To expand your Chair Walk, simply swing your arms or move your hands. There are lots of ways to do this. Swing your arms alternately and slowly with elbows slightly bent, as if walking. Or, bring your hands up to your shoulders and then down. Try squeezing and extending your fingers. Or simply *hold* your arms out sideways at shoulder height, if you can, left palm up, right palm down. This can be hard work. Exercise within your abilities. Let your BODs outbreath power every action while your tightened belly muscles protect your low back.

FEET are the body's foundation. When locked in shoes all day, feet become weak. Focused movement of unrestrained feet is really beneficial. For this exercise, called Crab Walk, you want to be seated with your shoes off and knees bent so that your feet are under your knees. Pretend that your toes are crabs. Curl your toes, lifting your arch off the floor. Then release the curl, letting your whole foot move forward an inch or two. Repeat this several times to the extent of your reach. Repeat with your other foot. If you are able, you can exercise both feet together. Crab Walking creates strong ankles because all muscles and ligaments from your toes wrap around your ankles.

Now it is your turn to create some of your own chair exercises. How about rolling your feet over a tennis or golf ball? How about putting a small beach ball between your legs and squeezing? How about pretending that you are a windmill or a steam engine or that you are dancing in your chair or reaching for the stars? Remember to maintain your posture to the best of your ability, keeping your head over your shoulders, and shoulders over your hips with your chest pushed out. This posture, along with the active, belly-tightening outbreath, promotes the health of your spine. BODs is all about playing. Use your imagination. Release the kid inside. Let the outbreath empower you.

WALKING, RUNNING, AND . . .

Once you have a feel for your BODs outbreath-inbreath rhythms, they will become the foundation of your exercise, whether walking, hiking, running, dancing, cycling, swimming, skiing, sitting in a chair, or doing activities of daily living.

I love to hike and cross-country ski, especially at high altitudes. When I was in my twenties, I thought that fast-paced daily running was the required preparation for my strenuous wilderness treks. Now, after forty years of daily walking, I know that a walking program is fine preparation for strenuous activities, even at 8,000 to 10,000 feet above sea level.

When I am preparing for a rigorous vacation, I become more diligent one to two months prior. I change my regular one-hour daily neighborhood walk, adding more hills, walking them as fast as I can continuously for a half hour, focused on BODs, of course. I also climb up and down flights of stairs whenever the opportunity arises. This prepares my lungs for the reduced air pressure at high altitudes. It's the way to acclimate more easily, avoid high-altitude sickness and sleep disturbances, and have energy to enjoy an active vacation.

SOCIAL WALKING AND FITNESS WALKING

These two kinds of walking — social walking and fitness walking — are both very important. Social walking is basically walking and talking with a buddy. If you are the listener, it is a good opportunity to use BODs. If you are the talker, tighten your belly muscles as you speak. When you pause at the end of a thought, let air in quickly and get right back to your conversation.

Fitness walking is solo walking — just you — not you and a friend, not you and your dog, not you and your iPod — just you. This is the opportunity to develop body, mind, and spirit harmony. You deserve some time each day simply to move your body, for a very good reason — your whole being loves it.

Physical work does not count as exercise. Even though I worked for twenty years as a wilderness guide, I still had to stay in shape so that I could scout five mountains in one week, then climb them again with clients the next week. I still needed time for myself. Work of any kind is innately stressful. Exercise in today's world is a means of staying fit and managing stress so that you can do your daily work effectively.

Here are some recommendations for stress-free walking. When you start your walk, take an inventory of your body. Check your posture. Are your ears over your shoulders, shoulders over your hips, hips over your feet, and chest out? This ideal posture is how your body works best. Before starting, orient yourself by doing a few BODs cycles of outbreath and inbreath.

As you walk or run, keep your head up. It weighs twelve to fifteen pounds. There is no need to look at your feet. This causes neck strain. The nervous system is equipped with reliable eye-foot coordination. Gaze out about 3 to 5 feet in front of you to scan the near distance for safe passage.

What do you do with your arms when walking or running? I suggest keeping your arms slightly bent at your sides with hands relaxed. Let your arms move forward and back gently, not briskly, to avoid centrifugal force that flings blood into your fingers, causing the blood to pool, making your fingers feel fat. I am not a fan of walking or running with hand or leg weights because they place extraordinary strain on joints. Plus, all this additional activity — multitasking — suggests that what you're already doing is not enough. This is simply not true.

STRATEGY ON HILLS

Do you avoid hills? This is where BODs rhythms are essential if you want to meet the challenge of enjoying hills, and reap the benefits. Not only will you need to change your pace, but also create a shorter breathing cycle to bring air into your lungs more frequently. Your goal when you complete the hill is to be able to speak — *if you have voice, you have breath.*

I like to zigzag walking up and down hills. This removes some of the steepness from the experience, placing less pressure on my leg joints. My preference is to hike a combination of flat and hilly terrain. I find it easier to hike six miles with ups and downs than six flat miles. A combination of terrain utilizes different muscles and prevents overuse, tiredness, and boredom.

DEALING WITH CRAMPS

During your exercise routine, you may experience cramps or spasms. When muscles do not receive adequate oxygen during exercise or daily activity, they become tense or tight. They may feel heavy. It becomes hard for oxygenated blood to flow through the muscle because of increased tension. BODs helps you to relax from the inside out and release tension so that oxygen can flow into the muscles.

Your job is to *stretch the cramping muscle*, just as you would uncoil a kinked garden hose. Place your hand on the cramping muscle as a means of identifying the spot that needs help. Then use your imagination to exhale into that place. If your calf muscle is cramping, bring your toes toward your knee to stretch the muscle as you exhale. If it's your shin that's cramping, point your toes down as you exhale.

There is another muscle that frequently cramps — the diaphragm, primary muscle of breathing. It's the saucer-shaped muscle under your ribs forming the floor of the chest cavity and roof of the abdomen. Runners, or people who do fast-paced exercise, and sedentary folks often complain of having a "stitch" (a cramp in the diaphragm), usually felt on the side of the body under the ribs. It's like a pinch. This is your diaphragm saying, "Ouch! I need more oxygen."

Use BODs to overcome this diaphragm cramping. If you have a stitch while using BODs, change your outbreath-inbreath rhythm to solve the problem so you don't have to slow down, stop, or quit. Create a slightly shorter outbreath to bring air into your lungs more frequently and satisfy your increased need for energy.

Nutritional Cramp Relief

When you have frequent cramps, the lacking nutrient is often potassium. Try eating a banana every now and then. If you continue to have cramps, even while using BODs appropriately and drinking adequate water, contact your health care provider because there are other causes of cramps.

Cool Down

After hard or extended exercise, you should continue to exercise at an easy pace—the cooldown—for at least a few minutes to lower your heart rate. This allows your leg muscles to continue pumping blood up to your heart while it's changing its rhythm, and to remove waste products like lactic acid from muscles. "If the heart has to do this work unaided by the leg-muscle pump, you are straining your heart to a point of failure," says Lee Coleman, professor emeritus of physical education at Whitman College, Walla Walla, Washington. "So cooling down starts the flushing-out process. If you wait or just stop, you will be sore."

Daily Water Intake

Drink plenty of water, all day long. Every organ in your body requires water for optimal function. Did you know that you lose more water via your lungs than via your kidneys? Water is the universal solvent that flushes toxins out of the body. These toxins, waste products of exercise and respiration, are normal. What's not normal and not healthy is for toxins to hang around in the body.

To determine the amount of water to drink, take your weight in pounds and divide it in half. This is the minimum number of ounces you should drink per day. The recommended average minimum is two quarts per day. If your water intake is inadequate, gradually increase your daily amount over a month or two to avoid feeling bloated. If you exercise regularly or are on medication, you need additional water.

Air and water are the two most important body requirements. Movement is the third element. Now that you know how to choreograph BODs with exercise, you're on the road to becoming your own personal trainer.

REALITY CHECK
EXPANDING YOUR BODs PRACTICE

1. What BODs techniques are you mastering?
2. What is your body teaching you?
3. How are you using BODs to enhance exercise and daily activities?

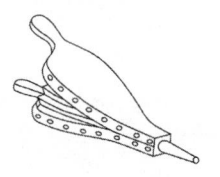

CHAPTER 7

CAREGIVERS AND BODs

Perfect Together

"Self-development is a higher duty than self-sacrifice."
Elizabeth Cady Stanton,
American women's rights activist

Helping others is part of the human experience. So actually, everyone is a caregiver. In fact, it is often easier to focus on helping others than on helping yourself—the caregiver's trap. However, in order to be of service, first you must maintain your own health and well-being. This requires a strong sense of self and an understanding that time spent on self-care is time well spent.

Caring for Yourself

I am always interested to know how people who work in health care take care of themselves, because *teaching by example is so powerful*. I want my colleagues and my own doctor to demonstrate excellent self-care. This engenders trust, a fundamental element of caring.

The way to be the best caregiver is to start with yourself. *Do your daily due diligence.* The BreatheOutDynamic system helps you get acquainted with your own body and learn to love it. BODs is the starting place for developing a cooperative relationship between your mind, your body, and your spirit.

Whether you work in a hospital transport department or on a surgical team, manage a home care company or care for a family member, being a caregiver is as stressful and demanding as it is rewarding. In order to do your daily work with a positive outlook, without being burdened by the pain of others, without feeling sorry for others, you must focus on your own health every day. It is time well spent—not lost—because you gain energy, efficiency, and clarity of purpose. The rewards are innumerable.

The BreatheOutDynamic system is a powerfully effective means to accomplish your personal focus on wellness. Here's why:

- BODs maximizes the extraordinary capabilities of breath, connecting each cell in your body and linking you with the environment beyond—the source of energy.
- BODs is fun to learn and easy to teach because it uses images like the bellows and pinwheel.

Muscles learn best when you envision the picture of a task.

- BODs can be incorporated into daily life, enabling everybody to benefit even when talking, giggling, laughing, humming, or grunting. The Seven Dwarfs must have been focused on BODs — whistling while they worked.

- BODs outbreath has a calming effect that makes you strong.

- BODs is cost effective. There is nothing to buy. All you have to spend is time — learning and using BODs.

- BODs is energy efficient because it utilizes natural forces like suction and gravity, and allows the diaphragm to do its most important work in a relaxed state. The result is less energy needed for breathing and more energy for living.

- BODs is nonjudgmental and introduces you to the art of listening to your own body's intelligence. It's not about breathing the right way. Rather, it's about you designing breathing cycles that are effective and efficient for *your* life.

- BODs presents you with the gift of self-knowledge, the gift of personal control, and the gifts of balance and well-being.

Now that you're taking good care of yourself, you're ready to care for others.

CARING FOR OTHERS

Once you are dedicated to practicing and using the BreatheOutDynamic system, you can use it while you are actually working, whether it is lifting a patient or equipment, drawing blood, suturing a wound, or wiping a brow.

You can also share BODs with the person you're caring for. It can be as easy as asking your patient to pretend to blow on a pinwheel. *Ta-dah!* BODs happens. Often, patients think that they are bystanders in the whole process of caring. Actually, they have an important role to play — that of being relaxed. *You cannot command someone to relax.*

True relaxation results from focusing on the BreatheOutDynamic system. For example: a relaxed, confident patient who practices BODs is much easier to transfer from bed to chair than an uptight, stressed out, passive one. BODs practiced by patient *and* caregiver rewards both.

The BreatheOutDynamic system pulls you out of the disease-management hole and engages you in the process of living, not the process of dying. When you are focused on living, every moment counts. When you are focused on dying, nothing matters — the past is more perfect than the present moment. BODs lets you experience this moment with joy or sadness, full of passion, not pity, without feeling sorry for yourself or others.

It's easy to be overcome by physical and psychic pain during illness. BODs guides you toward acceptance of this moment, this breath, without being troubled by the past or afraid of the future. BODs lets you reach deep into your inner resources to explore your energy reserves and to relax from the core. At a time when you may feel powerless, BODs keeps you involved in life.

REALITY CHECK
EXPANDING YOUR BODS PRACTICE

1. What is your commitment to self-care?
2. What BODs techniques help you manage stress?
3. How are you sharing BODs with others?

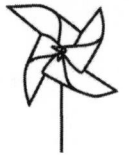

CHAPTER 8

ANSWERS TO FREQUENTLY ASKED QUESTIONS

"With a new day comes new strengths and thoughts."
Eleanor Roosevelt, First Lady
of the United States, 1933–1945
Chair, United Nations Commission
on Human Rights

LEARNING EFFECTIVE BREATHING THE BREATHEOUTDYNAMIC SYSTEM

1. WHY DON'T WE LEARN TO BREATHE MORE EFFECTIVELY AS CHILDREN?

SHORT ANSWER: School health curricula generally talk about breathing in a scientific way, without any practical application or training. In addition, textbooks define breathing as the process of taking *in* air. This action certainly pulls air into the lungs but is ineffective and inefficient.

LONG ANSWER: Actually, newborn babies know and use the BreatheOutDynamic system. As a fetus passes through the narrow birth canal, every organ in the about-to-be-born creature is squeezed. This is why a hearty cry is essential for the health of the newborn. The cry means that nature's vacuum is creating the suction required to overcome the collapsed nature of newborn lungs, now receiving air for the first time. After the very first inbreath, all human beings are using BODs. But at the same time, this unconscious breathing process in newborns starts to change as the baby's environment expands day by day, year to year.

Baby animals, including human beings, learn from their elders. Newborns learn from the people who hold them or scold them. This learning is transferred verbally and nonverbally. Most people in the United States — educators included — lack understanding of the personal effects of their own breathing. Thus, there is no awareness of the need to pay attention to the process of breathing. BODs is physical education at a deep, personal level.

As we grow through childhood, we are socialized to hold our breath or suck in air. Notice how adults respond to children when they are hurt. Adults often instruct children to stuff their feelings, saying, "Stop crying this minute," or "It's okay, no need to cry." This teaches kids or anyone to stop the outbreath (crying) and start sucking in air. Such instructions influence impressionable, growing human beings to store and personalize their anxieties — for a lifetime. Kids sniffle up their runny noses, wipe their eyes with the back of their hands, and take *in* short breaths as they try to accommodate adults' unspoken message: "Just get over it." Better to say, "Just blow on your pinwheel."

For further discussion, read Chapter 3, "Learn the BreatheOutDynamic system — The Two-Step Basics."

2. SINCE BREATHING IS UNCONSCIOUS, WHY SHOULD I CHANGE MY LIFELONG BREATHING HABITS?

SHORT ANSWER: If you would like to have more energy, be more relaxed, or resolve medical issues without medication or surgery, then it's worth your time and commitment to bring breathing into your consciousness. You do this by practicing the BreatheOutDynamic system.

For incentive from folks who already know and use BODs, read Chapter 1, "Inspiration from the Outbreath — BreatheOutDynamic system Stories."

LONG ANSWER: This book *is* the long answer.

3. DO I HAVE TO FOCUS ON THE BreatheOutDynamic SYSTEM ALL THE TIME?

SHORT ANSWER: No. Fortunately our bodies can bring in air without our conscious involvement. But, if you want to receive the benefits of the BreatheOutDynamic system, regular practice is essential.

LONG ANSWER: The more frequently you practice the BreatheOutDynamic system, the more your muscles respond and remember. Sit or lie down in a quiet place 3 times a day and focus on BODs for 5 to 15 minutes—

longer if you like. This is how you teach your muscles to understand BODs. Be right there with your body, experiencing how it responds. Become a dedicated BODs practitioner. Incorporate it into your daily activities, especially if you have difficulty breathing — for any reason.

For more ideas, read Chapter 6, "Becoming Your Own Personal Trainer."

4. WILL THE BreatheOutDynamic SYSTEM EVER BECOME MY UNCONSCIOUS BREATHING PROCESS?

SHORT ANSWER: With regular daily BODs practice over a long period of time, it is possible that your unconscious, default breathing will become BODs.

LONG ANSWER: As you read this book and practice BODs every day, you gain confidence that you have the ability to influence how your body works. This is a slow process, so be generous with your appreciation of what your body is achieving, and know that you can redesign your breathing.

Remember, you are learning something new, not undoing something you've been doing your whole life. The focus is on positive action, not negative thinking. Your body will thank you in so many ways. Enjoy the discovery.

5. WHAT IS THE DIFFERENCE BETWEEN BASIC BELLY BREATHING AND BODs?

SHORT ANSWER: Basic belly breathing engages belly muscles, also called abdominals or abs, to assist in moving the diaphragm, typically during both outbreath *and* inbreath. BODs engages abs during outbreath only. During BODs inbreath, abs are relaxed.

Long Answer: The difference between belly breathing and BODs is this: While belly breathing engages abs during both outbreath and inbreath, BODs engages the belly *only* during the outbreath. The BODs inbreath is passive and relaxed. That is, abs are relaxed to allow the diaphragm to descend, enlarging the lungs downward to create space for inrushing air. This significant decrease in your work of breathing — truly a net gain of energy — sets BODs apart from all other breathing methods.

To learn more, read Chapter 4, "How Your BODy Works — Rethinking Breathing."

6. Are there any problems associated with using the BreatheOutDynamic system?

Short Answer: There is one minor issue that sometimes appears when you first learn BODs. If you exhale too long or too forcefully, you might release too much carbon dioxide and thus feel light-headed or dizzy. To resolve this, simply cup your hands over your nose and mouth and rebreathe your exhaled air — until the dizziness disappears, usually in a moment or two. Continue using BODs with a slightly shorter outbreath.

Long Answer: In our blood, oxygen and carbon dioxide are circulating. The outbreath gathers carbon dioxide for its journey out of the body. The inbreath brings air from outside the body into the lungs where oxygen is extracted. The body maintains the right balance of these two blood gases in a series of interconnected processes that includes breathing. The light-headedness you might experience when first learning BODs tells you that there is not quite enough CO_2 remaining in your blood at the end of the outbreath. To resolve this, change your BODs rhythm by making your outbreath slightly shorter and less forceful. Your body will soon adjust to your more efficient BODs efforts.

To learn more, read Chapter 5, "The Next Step — Using BODs with Movement."

7. MY YOGA INSTRUCTOR TELLS ME TO BREATHE IN AND OUT ONLY THROUGH MY NOSE. WHY IS THE BreatheOutDynamic SYSTEM PROMOTING THE OUTBREATH THROUGH PURSED LIPS AND THE INBREATH THROUGH NOSE AND MOUTH?

SHORT ANSWER: Restricting the flow of air out of your mouth — by gently pursing your lips or using your teeth or tongue — helps to maintain an open airway, ensuring an adequate outbreath followed by an adequate inbreath, especially with activity.

LONG ANSWER: When Ian Jackson was developing BODs, he was approaching breathing from an athlete's point of view. Providing enough air to power athletic endeavors requires air to come in through nose *and* mouth. Applied to the general population and those with chronic illness, BODs focus on the active, spine-stretching, pursed-lipped outbreath and passive, relaxed inbreath through the mouth *and* the nose is appropriate and beneficial, and often necessary. For some people with chronic illness, even getting out of a chair is an athletic endeavor.

An eight-year-old boy at asthma camp asked me if it's possible to purse your nose. I had never thought of this. I suggested that he try it. I did too. What we discovered is that nose pursing is effective when using BODs while seated or lying down, but not when physically active, when the demand for oxygen is higher.

8. I HEAR MY EXERCISE INSTRUCTOR SAYING, "BREATHE FROM THE DIAPHRAGM." I KNOW WHERE THE DIAPHRAGM IS LOCATED, BUT I WONDER, "WHAT EXACTLY DOES THIS STATEMENT MEAN?"

SHORT ANSWER: Your instructor really means to *use* your diaphragm, but has not instructed you how to do this.

LONG ANSWER: The diaphragm, like the heart, is a muscle that we cannot consciously move. BODs active, spine-stretching outbreath compresses your guts up against your diaphragm and moves it up about one inch, pushing air out of your lungs. During BODs passive, relaxed inbreath, the diaphragm descends about one inch, stretching the lungs that are attached to it, pulling air into your lungs. This is what's happening when we are "breathing from the diaphragm," a statement that BODs instructors don't use, because you cannot consciously wiggle your diaphragm.

For more information, read Chapter 4, "How Your BODy Works — Rethinking Breathing."

9. IF I CAN'T USE MY BELLY MUSCLES, CAN I STILL USE THE BreatheOutDynamic SYSTEM?

SHORT ANSWER: Yes, here's how. Focus on gently restricting the flow of air as you blow out, like blowing on a pinwheel. Then simply do nothing for 1 or 2 seconds. During that time, your belly and diaphragm automatically relax and expand, inviting in air.

LONG ANSWER: Many people who think they can't use their belly muscles simply have weak belly muscles — most likely from disuse. To restore belly function, place a hand on your belly and push gently toward your spine during each outbreath. Release for each inbreath. Remember, effective muscle use is developed with practice.

One of my first respiratory home care patients with ALS (amyotrophic lateral sclerosis) taught me that even with muscle paralysis, you can benefit from BODs. Grace was totally paralyzed by ALS. Even with shortness of breath and a nonfunctioning diaphragm, she chose not to use a breathing machine. I assumed Grace could not use her belly muscles — after all, she was totally paralyzed. It was most difficult to communicate with her. She could grunt but could not speak. Then one day, it dawned on me that her grunt *was* her outbreath. Therefore Grace was actually engaging her belly muscles and using BODs. When we discussed this, she realized that she had a means to control her breath. Her belly muscles put her back in charge of one wee little aspect of her life. Grace lived for another few months and greeted me at each visit with a grunt and a smile.

Grace's success inspired me with another ALS patient, Joyce, who was using a mechanical ventilator 24/7 via a tracheostomy tube that bypassed her larynx (voice box). Thus she could not speak because air was not passing through her larynx. When I would take Joyce off her vent for a momentary, routine equipment check, her blood oxygen saturation dipped to 86% (97% and above is normal). I asked her to *pretend* to hum while off the vent. While doing this, the finger sensor showed her blood oxygen saturation stabilizing at 94%, adequate for an immobile person. Joyce was demonstrating the power of her imagination and outbreath.

10. I HEAR ABOUT SO MANY DIFFERENT WAYS TO BREATHE—LIKE YOGA AND BUTEYKO. HOW DO I KNOW WHAT'S RIGHT?

SHORT ANSWER: Try all breathing methods and observe the difference. Your body will tell you what works best. Just listen. Then choose your breathing method and incorporate it into your life.

LONG ANSWER: There is no right or wrong way to breathe. But there is an efficient and effective way to breathe. It's called the BreatheOutDynamic system, which is derived from yoga wisdom that says strength comes from the outbreath. The Buteyko breathing method, unlike BODs, recommends breath holding and is not designed for use with activities of daily living or for coordination with exercise. You decide what works for you.

11. I HAVE LUNG DISEASE. I LEARNED PURSED-LIP BELLY BREATHING IN MY PULMONARY REHABILITATION CLASS. WHAT'S THE DIFFERENCE BETWEEN THIS AND THE BreatheOutDynamic SYSTEM?

SHORT ANSWER: Pursed-lip belly breathing, while providing some benefits, relies on an active *in*breath during which you needlessly expend energy sucking *in* air.

LONG ANSWER: The BreatheOutDynamic system addresses both how to efficiently exhale and efficiently inhale, which results in major energy savings. People with little energy to begin with, such as those in pulmonary rehab, greatly benefit from this dynamic difference in methodology. For details, read Chapter 3, "Learn the BreatheOutDynamic system—The Two-Step Basics" and Chapter 4, "How Your BODy Works—Rethinking Breathing."

BENEFITS OF THE BREATHEOUTDYNAMIC SYSTEM

12. I LOVE TO HIKE, ESPECIALLY UP MOUNTAINS AT HIGH ALTITUDES. HOW CAN THE BREATHEOUTDYNAMIC SYSTEM HELP ME?

SHORT ANSWER: Use BODs every step of the way for energy and fullness of breath—as opposed to shortness of breath.

To get started, read Chapter 3, "Learn the BreatheOutDynamic system—The Two-Step Basics" and Chapter 5, "The Next Step—Using BODs with Movement."

LONG ANSWER: When I'm hiking or cross-country skiing at any altitude, my goal is to be comfortable in my body—no huffing and puffing along the way or at the top. And no need to stop to catch my breath. After decades of using BODs, my body is tuned in to varying terrains and the needs of each. Thus, it is important for you to pay attention to your smart body as well as where you are at the moment.

13. I'VE TRIED TO MEDITATE, BUT I CAN'T SIT STILL AND MY MIND WANDERS. CAN BODS HELP ME GAIN THE BENEFITS OF MEDITATION?

SHORT ANSWER: Yes. BODs can help you meditate and reap the benefits, and you don't even need to be seated. Coordinating the BreatheOutDynamic system with activity, such as walking, is moving meditation.

Read Chapter 5, "The Next Step—Using BODs with Movement."

Long Answer: Meditation is a focus on this very moment. When concentrating on BODs, you are totally absorbed in the present moment. Because most of your BODs energy is directed toward the outbreath, relaxation occurs deep within your body. You don't need to worry about your mind wandering because your mind is totally absorbed in counting steps as you walk. Your mind and your body are working together—moving meditation. Ironically, even after activity, you will feel relaxed, energized, and refreshed.

14. I'm pregnant. Will the BreatheOutDynamic system help me manage pain when giving birth?

Short Answer: Yes. BODs minimizes all sorts of pain. You'll benefit most by sharing BODs with someone who can coach you during the birthing process.

Long Answer: BODs is a breathing system for a myriad of needs in all aspects of your life—for relaxation, stress and pain management, strength enhancement, and energy conservation. Start using BODs early in your pregnancy to provide good oxygen flow for you and your baby, as well as a wonderful massage.

Then, during the stress of labor and delivery, concentrate on the outbreath when your uterus is contracting. Thus your strong abdominal muscles will support the work of your uterus. Between contractions, focus on your BODs rhythm with help from your coach.

After delivery, use BODs to help your abdominal

muscles return to normal function and promote the relaxation required for breastfeeding. In addition, your baby will be absorbing BODs rhythms through your body. What a great start you're providing.

For more information, refer to Chapter 5, "The Next Step—Using BODs with Movement."

15. CAN THE BreatheOutDynamic SYSTEM HELP IN THE HEAT OF INTERCOURSE?

SHORT ANSWER: Sure. Try it.

LONG ANSWER: Using BODs during sexual activity energizes and relaxes you safely at a time when your muscles are working hard and when relaxation is essential for optimum orgasms—whether for pleasure or procreation.

THE BreatheOutDynamic SYSTEM AND THE UNKNOWN

16. HOW DO I KNOW THAT AIR HAS ACTUALLY ENTERED MY LUNGS IF I DON'T INHALE?

SHORT ANSWER: You must learn to *trust* that all the air you push out comes right back in because *you* create a vacuum with your active, spine-stretching outbreath.

LONG ANSWER: Have you ever played with a toy mouse, the kind that squeaks when you squeeze the air out of it? Have you ever used an oven baster to gather pan drippings to make gravy? These are two examples of how BODs works. Here's the physics: If you squeeze something, then suddenly let it expand, you create a vacuum/suction that sucks in the gas or liquid—sometimes even a solid, as in choking. With the mouse and oven baster, you never question that air and pan drippings enter. It always works this way—even when the container is your lungs. This is why trust is so important.

To learn more about the physics of air entering automatically with the passive inbreath, read Chapter 2, "Building the Case for the BreatheOutDynamic system—Proof Is in Your BODy."

17. Why has the BreatheOutDynamic system been such a well-kept secret?

Short Answer: There is no short answer.

Long Answer: Historically, the active outbreath has been an esoteric art, used exclusively by the ruling class in martial arts. The common person had no access to this knowledge. Starting in the 1960s, Ian Jackson adapted this ancient wisdom about strength and relaxation for use with continuous activities like walking and cycling. He intentionally made BODs freely available to all. Your BODs practice fulfills his intention.

Health care in the twentieth century led us on a path that included dependence on medication and surgery for health maintenance. Now in the twenty-first century, awareness is building regarding the benefits of effective breathing and daily exercise for well-being. You are invited to be part of this healthy change.

THE BREATHEOUTDYNAMIC SYSTEM LIVING WITH DYSFUNCTION

18. I HAD PART OF MY LUNGS REMOVED. NOW MY SPEECH IS AFFECTED. HOW CAN THE BREATHEOUTDYNAMIC SYSTEM HELP ME?

SHORT ANSWER: In order to have voice, you need *out*breath — air flowing over your vocal cords during expiration. BODs is perfect for this assignment.

LONG ANSWER: Here's why your voice may be weaker after lung surgery: 1) Surgery removed part of your lungs. Thus you have less air to expel for voice projection. 2) During surgery you were intubated — an endotracheal tube was passed through your vocal cords. A breathing machine was connected to the end of the tube hanging out of your mouth. After surgery you were extubated — the tube was pulled out. Intubation and extubation may have damaged your vocal cords. Healing can take many months. BODs practice will not only help you project your voice, it will also rest your vocal cords, prevent overuse, and help them heal.

19. I HAVE ASTHMA. HOW CAN THE BREATHEOUTDYNAMIC SYSTEM HELP?

SHORT ANSWER: Asthma is tightness of airway muscles

with multiple causes, not the least of which are negative emotions and stress. BODs active, spine-stretching outbreath stimulates the nervous system to help all muscles relax from the inside out. Relaxation is essential, especially when there is a crisis. Additionally, BODs focus on the active outbreath helps to keep your airway open. To overcome the effects of asthma, become committed to the BreatheOutDynamic system. Also, do your own research to learn more about the health of your whole body.

Long Answer: Have you ever wondered why people with asthma who use their medications as prescribed still have asthma attacks and die? Here's one possibility: Medication simply masks the symptoms, as well as the causes, of breathing problems, which are lumped into the term "asthma." The National Institutes of Health recommends that people with asthma keep a log of their symptoms for more effective drug use, but never suggests documenting their state of being or using nondrug approaches, such as the BreatheOutDynamic system.

Whenever your airway is blocked, fear takes over. Or perhaps fear caused the blockage. Chronic airway blockage releases a cascade of hormones, which creates more stress and muscle tightness, affecting every organ in your body. During an asthma attack, the harder you try to take *in* a breath, the worse the breathlessness becomes.

Here's what I recommend to decrease your

dependence on quick-acting, rescue-medicine inhalers —
albuterol or Proventil. Do NOT use a rescue inhaler
whenever you feel short of breath. Instead, sit down and
focus on BODs for 5 to 15 minutes to relax your entire
body. Then, reassess your need for rescue medication. In
most cases, your shortness of breath will be gone because
you relaxed with BODs.

If you are using a steroid inhaler — a totally
different kind of medicine — understand that it is not
"rescue" medicine. Steroid medication must always be
used on schedule, as prescribed, or it won't work. Keep
your doctor informed about your progress.

I am a respiratory therapist, not a medical doctor;
thus I cannot prescribe drugs. Rather, I recommend BODs.
My professional responsibility is to ensure that prescribed
medications and recommended therapies are safe and
appropriate. I have witnessed the overprescribing of
rescue medications for anyone who reports shortness
of breath. Health is achieved by discovering causes
and taking appropriate actions rather than covering up
the symptoms with medication. Doctors, respiratory
therapists, nurses, and patients all need to work together
to optimize health safely.

I recommend that people with asthma educate
themselves about how the human body functions and
be fastidious about daily self-care — nutritious foods,

adequate water intake, relaxation, stress management, and daily exercise using BODs. Ask your doctor for help to reduce your need for medication or connect with a doctor who sees beyond medication and beyond lungs to the whole person.

One caution: If BODs is to be effective in times of need, it must be learned and practiced every day. Do not expect to be saved by a system that you have simply *read* about or that none of the significant people in your life know about and actually use. Consider asking a buddy to join you in your BODs practice.

20. I HAVE CHRONIC OBSTRUCTIVE PULMONARY DISEASE (COPD). HOW CAN THE BREATHEOUTDYNAMIC SYSTEM HELP MY SHORTNESS OF BREATH?

SHORT ANSWER: People with COPD have difficulty exhaling adequate air because increased air pressure in their lungs restricts movement of the diaphragm, the most important muscle of respiration. Some of this problem is overcome with BODs focus on the active outbreath, using the contents of the belly to push up against the diaphragm. You must learn BODs and use it routinely for it to be of service to you.

LONG ANSWER: COPD makes Swiss cheese of lung tissue, which loses its elasticity. Then mucus rushes in to protect damaged tissue—a normal response. But all this mucus can ultimately create shortness of breath. Also, air is trapped in the lungs and cannot get out, adding air pressure that pushes down on the diaphragm, forcing it to work hard to overcome resistance. Over time, the diaphragm flattens out and is disabled. Because BODs engages belly muscles to aid the diaphragm, it is an appropriate protocol for people with COPD or any lung dysfunction. Be sure to share your BODs practice with your doctor and your respiratory therapist.

21. CAN THE BREATHEOUTDYNAMIC SYSTEM HELP WITH PAIN MANAGEMENT?

SHORT ANSWER: Absolutely.

LONG ANSWER: When you experience pain of any kind — whether from illness or injury or when you're in the dentist's chair — your body becomes tense. Think of tense as meaning tight, or intense, or magnified. All muscles have the potential to tighten up, especially the ones you can't see. Thus, blood pressure increases and arterial blood flow decreases. Nerves that are compressed by tight muscles can cause tingling and numbness, or pain and immobility. BODs relaxes muscles so pain becomes less intense. When in pain, it's difficult to remember how to help yourself. It is essential to learn and use BODs routinely with all activity every day so that when you need help, your body and mind can work together.

To learn from the experiences of others,

read Chapter 1, "Inspiration from the Outbreath—BreatheOutDynamic system Stories."

I hope these questions and answers have intrigued you to learn and question more.

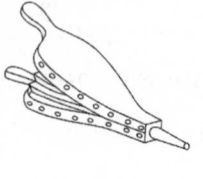

EPILOGUE

BODs Bonus
FINDING YOUR INNER VOICE:
CONNECTING BODY, MIND, AND SPIRIT

"Be empty, and you will remain full."
Lao-Tsu, Chinese philosopher

"I found the greatest love of all inside of me."
Whitney Houston, singer, songwriter

In the twenty-first century, the inner voice — the soul's expression — is drowning in the din and distraction of electronics. Television is used as a stimulant and sedative. We place babies in front of it. We eat with our eyes glued to it. We let television lull us into boredom and then sleep, only to be woken up by a computer voice reciting the time or an electronic bird chirping. Whatever happened to daylight and sunshine?

Electronic gadgets consume our imagination. While driving, we talk to someone who is not in the car and listen to an electronic voice telling us where to go.

With all this input, there is no time or space for output — your inner voice, your creative expression, your intuition. We are stuck in a quagmire of noise — visual and auditory — blind to the possibilities.

To find your inner voice, you have to know what to listen for. Only you can hear it. It's the essential you — the fun-loving, creative, passionate being. Your inner voice is heard by you — not by your parents, siblings, spouse, friends, or colleagues. In the process of growing up, it often gets squelched in a thick coating of parental commands that include words like should-a, could-a, would-a. This thick crud can include power plays and sexual misconduct. Thus, the volume dial on your adult inner voice could be turned really low, or even broken. You may have truly lost your inner voice, which you had as a kid. Take a symbolic visit back to your childhood to find that essential, fun-loving you.

There are several stages to opening the door to your inner voice. First, you must love your body unconditionally. This represents your acceptance of your body as it is at this moment. Self-love is available to all who breathe regardless of physical attributes or abilities. Let's face it: no one's body is perfect. This lack of perfection can make it easier to leap into acceptance because acceptance is simply an attitude, not a list of characteristics.

An attitude is a thought, often expressed by action.

You are in charge of your attitudes. So, embrace your body, literally. Put your arms around yourself and say these words out loud: "I love my body, my representation to the world of who I am."

That's it! That's how simple it can be. If you don't accept all your foibles and inconsistencies, you will project that disdain onto others who are completely innocent of your deception.

Loving your body includes taking care of those foibles that may be hindering your life. You can make those important changes only in the presence of self-love, the key to personal motivation. Change can happen in your lifetime—just be aware that it's a slow process but well worth the investment of your time and energy.

The second stage of opening the door to your inner voice is to develop a user-friendly body. The key word is develop, which refers to the ongoing actions you take every day to encourage your body to be the best it can be. This would include how you breathe, what you eat, drink, and inhale, how you move, how you manage stress, and what you do for fun.

The BreatheOutDynamic system is a significant part of developing a user-friendly body because BODs brings oxygen, essential for full function, to every cell in your body. Since every cell is connected to every other cell, BODs creates a cascade effect. When muscles and organs are nourished with adequate oxygen, movement becomes joyful. The mind chatter of pain, stiffness, or exhaustion quiets down. The din of disuse is replaced by the musings of your inner voice. This is truly meditation—a BODs bonus.

Here's an activity that engages your inner voice. Suppose you have an important decision to make. You've been thinking about it for days—this is brain work. Now, let's engage your body to access your inner voice, which can assist in the decision-making process. This involves taking a walk for thirty minutes or so. Prior to setting out, generate a yes-no question in your head, related to your important decision. Then go for your walk. Use BODs and enjoy your surroundings. *Do not think about the question while walking.* Upon returning, ask yourself the original question. Then immediately ask for the answer. It's either *yes* or *no.* Your body will instantly, without prejudice, tell you the answer. You'll know it's correct because you will experience deep contentment.

The third stage of your search for your inner intelligence is to discover activities that bring you joy: dancing, kneading bread, restoring old things, riding a bike or horse, growing plants, whistling, sharing your expertise. With your brain and body content, you will hear your inner voice loud and clear.

Finding your inner voice is a worthwhile project that you will never regret. It requires silence so that you can listen and trust that your life and breath can evolve by your own design. Having read this book, you've started your journey. Now with *Just Breathe Out* as your guidebook, continue on your way using the revolutionary BreatheOutDynamic system.

Best wishes on your BODs journey—and please, do send a postcard.

Happy trails!

Send your postcard to Betsy Thomason at betsy@justbreatheout.com.

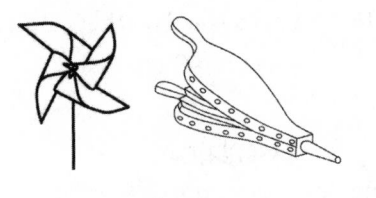

List of Illustrations
Alice Goldsmith, illustrator

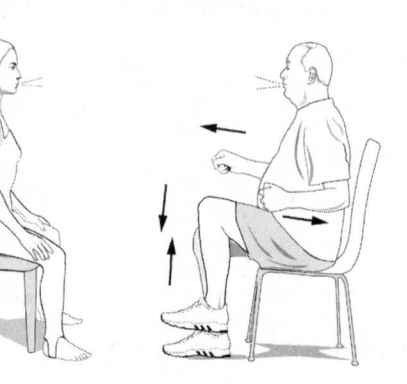

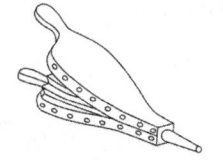

PINWHEEL
TEMPLATE AND INSTRUCTIONS

MATERIALS

- scissors
- small piece of clear tape
- pushpin
- pencil with eraser

DIRECTIONS

- Tear this page out of the book and cut out the square, or create your own square on a separate piece of paper.
- Cut to the end of the dotted lines, stopping about an inch from the center.
- Gently bend (do NOT fold) every other point so that the tips overlap the center and each other.
- Tape the points in place.
- Push the pin through the overlapping tips and the center of the pinwheel.
- Push the pin into the top of the pencil eraser, leaving room for the pinwheel to spin.

Now you have a tool to practice your outbreath and
see its amazing power.

Thanks to pinwheelsforpeace.com for the template.

If every body experiences peace, everybody will be at peace.

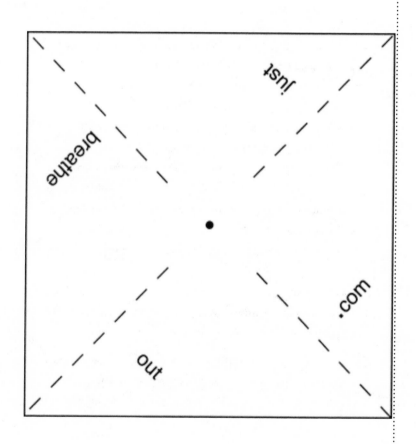

just
breathe
out
.com

the BreatheOutDynamic system the BreatheOutDynamic system
www.justbreatheout.com www.justbreatheout.com
the BreatheOutDynamic system the BreatheOutDynamic system

the BreatheOutDynamic system the BreatheOutDynamic system
www.justbreatheout.com www.justbreatheout.com
the BreatheOutDynamic system the BreatheOutDynamic system

the BreatheOutDynamic system the BreatheOutDynamic system
www.justbreatheout.com www.justbreatheout.com
the BreatheOutDynamic system the BreatheOutDynamic system

the BreatheOutDynamic system the BreatheOutDynamic system
www.justbreatheout.com www.justbreatheout.com
the BreatheOutDynamic system the BreatheOutDynamic system

the BreatheOutDynamic system the BreatheOutDynamic system
www.justbreatheout.com www.justbreatheout.com
the BreatheOutDynamic system the BreatheOutDynamic system

About the Author

When Betsy Thomason graduated from American University in 1966 and accepted a teaching job in Spring Valley, New York, she knew of its proximity to Harriman State Park. What she didn't know was how powerful her outdoor adventures would be in shaping her future. Learning how to get up mountains without huffing and puffing put her in touch with people who introduced her to the power of the outbreath. Subsequently, she attended Bergen Community College and received an associate degree in respiratory therapy. Betsy credits her love for the outdoors with expanding the knowledge and experiences that she shares with others. She welcomes you to share your story with her at betsy@justbreatheout.com.

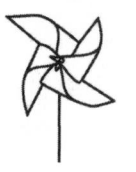